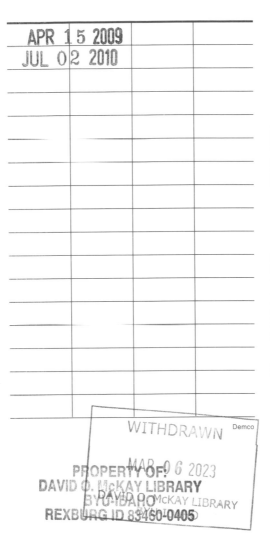

Strength Training
for Seniors

An Instructor Guide for Developing Safe and Effective Programs

Wayne L. Westcott, PhD, CSCS
South Shore YMCA
Quincy, MA

Thomas R. Baechle, EdD, CSCS, NSCA-CPT
Creighton University
Omaha, NE

Human Kinetics

Library of Congress Cataloging-in-Publication Data

Westcott, Wayne L., 1949-
    Strength training for seniors: an instructor guide for developing safe and effective
programs / Wayne L. Westcott, Thomas R. Baechle.
        p. cm.
    Includes bibliograhical references and index.
    ISBN 0-87322-952-5
    1. Physical fitness for the aged. 2. Physical education for the
aged. 3. Exercise for the aged--Physiological aspects. 4. Weight
training. 5. Muscle strength. I. Baechle, Thomas R., 1943-   .
II. Title.
    RA781.W42 1999   98-27028
    613.7'0446--dc21   CIP

ISBN: 0-87322-952-5

Acquisitions Editor: Loarn Robertson; **Developmental Editor:** Elaine Mustain; **Assistant
Editors:** Phil Natividad, Melissa Feld; **Copyeditor:** Brian C. Mustain; **Proofreader:** Jane
Hilken; **Indexer:** Craig Brown; **Graphic Designer:** Robert Reuther; **Graphic Artist:** Yvonne
Winsor; **Photo Editor:** Boyd LaFoon; **Cover Designer:** Jack Davis; **Photographer (cover):**
Tom Roberts; **Photographers (interior):** pp. 36-37, 155, 156 (top), 176, and 178 © by Melissa
Andronico; pp. 67, 93, 119, 158, and 168-170 © by Ford Jacobsen; p. 124 © by Nautilus; pp. 157
(top) and 193 © by Human Kinetics/Tom Roberts; All others © by Sharon Townson; **Illustra-
tors:** Tom Roberts, Tim Offenstein, Katherine Galasyn-Wright; **Printer:** Edwards Bros.

Printed in the United States of America   10 9 8 7 6 5 4 3 2 1

Human Kinetics
Web site: http://www.humankinetics.com/

United States: Human Kinetics
P.O. Box 5076
Champaign, IL 61825-5076
1-800-747-4457
e-mail: humank@hkusa.com

Canada: Human Kinetics
475 Devonshire Road Unit 100
Windsor, ON N8Y 2L5
1-800-465-7301 (in Canada only)
e-mail: humank@hkcanada.com

Europe: Human Kinetics, P.O. Box IW14
Leeds LS16 6TR, United Kingdom
(44) 1132 781708
e-mail: humank@hkeurope.com

Australia: Human Kinetics
57A Price Avenue
Lower Mitcham, South Australia 5062
(088) 277-1555
e-mail: humank@hkaustralia.com

New Zealand: Human Kinetics
P.O. Box 105-231, Auckland 1
(09) 523 3462
e-mail: humank@hknewz.com

We are privileged to dedicate this book to our wives, Claudia Westcott and Susan Baechle.

Contents

Acknowledgments

As the authors, this is the most satisfying page in our book, for we acknowledge with great appreciation some of the remarkable individuals who assisted us in producing this text. We begin with the most helpful staff at Human Kinetics, especially Ted Miller, Elaine and Brian Mustain, Loarn Robertson, Michael Bahrke, Melissa Feld, and Craig Newsom. We are also grateful for our fine photographers, Sharon Townson, Melissa Andronico, and Ford Jacobsen, as well as our highly cooperative exercise models, Edyce Binder, Diane Caledonia, Dick Carey, Robert Concannon, George Conway, Dr. Robert Creek, Ian Dargin, Marie Hegerty, Herb Kirshnit, Elaine Mustain, Fran Ramsden, Velma Sutherland, Verna Trotman, Skip Tull, and Warren Westcott. In addition, we thank Debra Wein, MS, RD, for her sound advice on healthy eating when strength training, and Steve Block, President of SPRI Products, Inc., for providing the resistance bands for the alternative strength exercise photos. Our special appreciation goes to the Executive Directors of the South Shore YMCA, Ralph Yohe, Mary Moore, and William Johnson and to the Director of Strength and Conditioning at Creighton University, Charlie Oborny, CSCS, NSCA-CPT. For their hours of typing and writing assistance, we gratefully acknowledge our secretaries, Susan Ramsden and Linda Tranisi. Most of all we appreciate the support of our wives, Claudia Westcott and Susan Baechle, as well as God's grace in making this writing project such an enjoyable and educational endeavor for us.

Introduction

During the past several years, researchers have discovered that many of the degenerative diseases and most of the general weakness that accompanies the aging process are related to loss of muscle mass and strength (Evans and Rosenberg 1992). Although a certain amount of strength attenuation is inevitable, numerous studies have shown that senior adults can maintain and regain muscle mass and strength at any age (Campbell et al. 1994; Westcott and Guy 1996). Postmenopausal women (Nelson et al. 1994), older men (Frontera et al. 1988), and even nonagenarians (Fiatarone et al. 1990) have all improved their musculoskeletal structure and function through relatively simple programs of strength training.

While most of the research has been conducted at universities, older adult strength training programs are currently provided by nursing homes, retirement villages, community centers, YMCAs, health clubs, and other organizations. The research results are remarkable—strength exercise has produced improved muscular fitness (Westcott and Guy 1996), increased metabolic rate (Campbell et al. 1994), increased bone mineral density (Menkes et al. 1993), enhanced gastrointestinal transit (Koffler et al. 1992), greater glucose utilization (Hurley 1994), better balance (Nelson et al. 1994), reduced low-back pain (Risch et al. 1993), decreased arthritic discomfort (Tufts 1994), and higher levels of self-confidence (Westcott 1995). Yet no clearly defined exercise protocol exists for older adult strength training.

The purpose of this book is to provide instructors of older adults with research-based principles for safe and successful strength training programs. Because putting principles into practice is your responsibility as the instructor, we have included chapters on general guidelines for senior strength training, specific teaching strategies and training procedures, standard free-weight and machine exercises, sample free-weight and machine workout programs, alternative exercises using bodyweight and elastic bands, practical methods for assessing progress, important information for training special populations, and nutrition for senior weight trainers.

To ensure proper performance of the strength exercises, this text features precise illustrations and detailed explanations of numerous machine, free-weight, bodyweight, and elastic band training exercises. We also describe procedures that you can use to systematically assess your older clients' training progress and to compare their progress with normative data in areas of leg strength, hip-trunk flexibility, and body composition.

One of the most useful features of this textbook is up-to-date information on the health and fitness benefits of strength training for mature men and women, as well as key considerations for instructing several special populations. These populations include those who suffer from obesity, diabetes, cardiovascular disease, osteoporosis, low-back pain, arthritis, depression, visual and auditory impairments, as well as general frailty.

Because more and more adults are realizing that muscles are the engines of their bodies and are beginning to experiment with strength training, the need for qualified professional instructors continues to increase. By studying the information presented in this book, you will acquire a better understanding of sensible strength training and gain confidence in presenting appropriate strength workouts to older adults. If you use the standard strength principles, implement the recommended exercise protocols, and follow the sample program designs, you will be able to provide effective leadership for senior strength training participants. The logical and progressive manner in which this information is presented makes it easy to comprehend and apply, with appropriate adaptations for your particular training situation. You should find the figures, tables, and logs especially helpful in setting up specific exercise programs and making strength training relevant to previously sedentary clients.

A successful strength training program can make the difference between older adults who have low strength levels and endure a sedentary existence, and those who have high strength levels and enjoy a physically active lifestyle. The tools in this textbook will enhance your skill as a professional strength training instructor and enable you to become a productive agent of change for the health of older adults in your community.

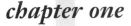

chapter one

Why Your Clients Should Train

Put yourself in the position of a typical older adult, say a 55-year-old male or female who has been physically inactive and has added 30 pounds of fat. You have been on several diets, but none has produced permanent reductions in bodyweight. You have tried walking, but your exercise schedule has been inconsistent and your body composition has remained essentially the same.

You have read a few articles about the benefits of strength training, and even glanced at a book on strength training for older adults. However, you're not fully convinced that this type of exercise can help you lose weight, and you've heard that it can actually raise your blood pressure. You're not very athletic and you've never even tried to lift weights. You're concerned about looking uncoordinated or experiencing an injury, and you're wondering if the benefits of strength training are really worth the effort.

Chances are, unless someone clearly explains why you should do strength training and carefully shows you how to perform the exercises properly, you are unlikely to attempt this unfamiliar physical activity. A fitness professional who is knowledgeable about strength training for older adults can play a vital role in helping you—along with a large segment of our population—get on track with respect to musculoskeletal fitness. In fact, research shows that strength training has many health and fitness applications beyond building stronger muscles.

This chapter presents the beneficial effects of strength training—including replacing muscle, reducing fat, increasing metabolic rate, decreasing low-back discomfort, relieving arthritic pain, preventing osteoporosis, enhancing glucose utilization, speeding up gastrointestinal transit, lowering resting blood pressure, improving blood lipid levels, and improving postcoronary performance, as well as boosting self-confidence and beating depression. This information should help you to sell older adults on the importance of strength training.

Body Composition

Most people realize that strength training is the best way to develop larger and stronger muscles. They know that bodybuilders do strength exercise to build exceptionally large muscles, and that weightlifters do strength exercise to lift exceptionally heavy weights. Because most older adults have no desire to compete in bodybuilding or weightlifting events, they tend to avoid strength training altogether. This is unfortunate because everyone, especially people over age 50, can benefit from larger and stronger muscles. Moreover, few people have the genetic potential to develop really large muscles, and those who do must work very deliberately to achieve exaggerated physiques, so fears of becoming too big or too strong are totally unfounded.

Too Little Muscle, Too Much Fat

In fact, the situation for almost all men and women is exactly the opposite. Rather than being concerned about too much muscle, they should be concerned about too little muscle. Adults who do not perform regular strength exercise lose about one-half pound of muscle per year during their 30s and 40s (Evans and Rosenberg 1992). Unfortunately, there is evidence that the rate of muscle loss doubles (one pound per year) in people over 50 years of age (Nelson et al. 1994). Even more disturbing, the number of Type II (fast-twitch) muscle fibers in sedentary males decreases more than 50% by age 80 (Larsson 1983). It is these fibers that are most involved in movements requiring high levels of strength. Because muscles are the engines of the body, this loss in muscle tissue is similar to dropping from an eight-cylinder engine to a four-cylinder engine, while the weight of the automobile keeps getting heavier.

Muscle loss causes two of life's major problems, and is associated with a variety of health-related consequences:

1. Reduced functional capacity, which leads to less physical activity and further muscle loss

2. Reduced calorie utilization, which leads to a slower metabolism and fat accumulation

Less muscle and more fat contributes to many degenerative diseases, including heart disease and diabetes. Most people realize that too much fat is a serious health threat, and many try to solve this problem through dieting. Unfortunately, even though at present 4 out of 10 Americans are dieting (Tufts 1992), fewer than 5% will be successful (Brehm and Keller 1990). This is because too much fat is only part of the problem, and losing fat is only part of the solution.

Gaining Muscle, Losing Fat

The less obvious but more important problem is too little muscle, and adding muscle is a double solution because it increases both physical capacity (a larger engine) and metabolic rate (higher energy requirements). Research shows that strength training can replace muscle (Grimby et al. 1992; McCartney et al. 1996) and increase metabolic rate (Campbell et al. 1994; Pratley et al. 1994) in older adults.

Consider the results of a recent study at Tufts University (Campbell et al. 1994) in which previously sedentary men and women (ages 56 to 80 years) performed approximately 30 minutes of relatively high-effort strength training (three sets each of five machine exercises) three days per week, for 12 weeks. At the end of the three-month training period, the participants had added about three pounds of lean weight, lost about four pounds of fat weight, and increased their resting metabolism by almost 7%. Doing about 90 minutes of strength training a week enabled these older adults to replace about three pounds of muscle, reduce about four pounds of fat, and eat significantly more calories per day in the process.

Unlike dieting, which decreases the number of calories eaten per day, strength training increases the number of calories used per day. But there are many other body composition benefits attained from a regular program of strength exercise.

Consider the results of a large-scale study (Westcott and Guy 1996) that examined the effects of strength and endurance exercise on young, middle, and older adults. The 1,132 men and women performed about 25 minutes of relatively high-effort strength training (one set each of 12 machine exercises) and 20 minutes of moderate-effort aerobic activity (treadmill walking or stationary cycling) two or three days a week for eight weeks. As shown in table 1.1, all three age categories added over 2 pounds of lean weight and lost over 4 pounds of fat weight. Note that the 60- to 80-year-old exercisers gained just as much muscle as the middle-aged and younger adults.

In a similar study (Westcott 1997), 69 older adults (mean age 56 years) performed relatively high-effort strength training alone (one set each of 12 machine exercises) three days a week for eight weeks. The subjects added 3.9 pounds of lean weight and lost 4.2 pounds of fat weight, for an eight-pound improvement in body composition.

A study by Butts and Price (1994) examined the effects of relatively high-effort strength training on body composition in women between 30 and 63 years of age. The participants completed one set each of 12 machine exercises,

Table 1.1

Changes in Body Weight and Body Composition for Young, Middle-Aged, and Older Program Participants (N = 1132)

Age	Body Wt. Pre (lb)	Body Wt. Post (lb)	Body Wt. Change (lb)	Body Fat Pre (%)	Body Fat Post (%)	Body Fat Change (%)	Fat Wt. Pre (lb)	Fat Wt. Post (lb)	Fat Wt. Change (lb)	Lean Wt. Pre (lb)	Lean Wt. Post (lb)	Lean Wt. Change (lb)
21-40 years (N = 238)	176.5	173.9	−2.6*	27.2	24.9	−2.3*	49.1	44.2	−4.9*	127.4	129.7	+2.3*
41-60 years (N = 553)	179.9	177.9	−2.0*	27.0	24.9	−2.1*	48.9	44.5	−4.4*	130.8	133.1	+2.3*
61-80 years (N = 341)	172.7	171.0	−1.7*	25.6	23.6	−2.0*	44.7	40.6	−4.1*	128.0	130.4	+2.4*

* Statistically significant change (p < .01)

three days a week for 12 weeks. The women increased their lean weight by 2.9 pounds and decreased their fat weight by 3.0 pounds.

Differences in muscle gain and fat loss may be due in part to gender specific responses to strength exercise. For example, in Westcott and Guy's 1996 study, on average the 749 female subjects added 1.7 pounds of lean weight and lost 3.4 pounds of fat weight, whereas the 383 male subjects added 3.7 pounds of lean weight and lost 6.4 pounds of fat weight. However, the key and consistent finding in these and other studies (Fiatarone et al. 1990; Frontera et al. 1988; Nelson et al. 1994) is that strength training is an effective means for improving body composition (both increasing lean weight and decreasing fat weight) in older adults.

Metabolic Rate

Muscle is very active tissue that requires large amounts of energy during exercise and a significant energy supply at rest. In the study by Campbell et al. (1994), 12 weeks of strength training produced a three-pound increase in lean weight and a 7% increase in resting metabolic rate in the older adult participants (figure 1.1). Whether the faster resting metabolism is due to more muscle tissue, more active muscle tissue, or both is not fully understood. However, it seems clear that the higher resting metabolisms in this and in a similar study by Pratley et al. (1994), that showed a 7.7% metabolic increase, were in response to the strength training programs. According to Paffenbarger and Olsen (1996), adding 10 pounds of muscle through strength training increases the daily resting energy requirements by about 500 calories.

In addition to the 7% increase in resting metabolism, participants in the Campbell et al. (1994) study had significantly greater daily energy requirements. Although they did not gain bodyweight, the subjects consumed approximately 15% more calories per day during the last two weeks of the study than they had during the first two weeks. The researchers attributed the increased caloric needs to both the higher resting metabolism and the energy cost of strength exercise.

Another metabolic effect of strength training is elevated postexercise energy expenditure. Research by Gillette et al. (1994) showed significantly higher energy utilization for 90 minutes following strength exercise as compared to endurance exercise, and Melby et al. (1993) found a 12% increase in metabolism two hours after a high-volume and high-intensity strength training workout. Although standard senior strength training sessions are unlikely to produce metabolic increases of this magnitude, they undoubtedly increase the participants' postexercise metabolic rates over resting levels.

Strength training appears to have a threefold effect on metabolic function: it produces a large increase in metabolic rate during the exercise session, a moderate increase in metabolic rate during the postexercise recovery period, and a small increase in resting metabolism throughout the day. Clearly, developing more muscle tissue and maintaining more active muscle tissue

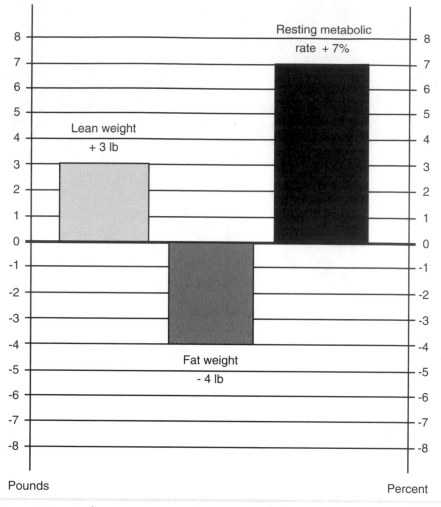

Figure 1.1 Body composition and resting metabolic rate changes in senior exercisers after 12 weeks of strength training (Campbell et al. 1994).

through regular strength training can effectively increase metabolic rate and energy utilization.

Back Pain

Although it sounds too bad to be true, medical professionals estimate that four out of five American adults experience low-back pain. In fact, this problem causes more employee absenteeism than any other illness or injury except for the common cold. Research (Jones et al. 1988) has shown a strong positive relationship between low-back discomfort and weak low-back muscles. A 12-year study at the University of Florida Medical School indicates that systematic strengthening of the low-back (trunk extension) muscles significantly reduces or eliminates pain in the majority of patients (Risch et al. 1993). Apparently, strong low-back muscles reduce stress in the spinal area, and prevent excessive wear and tear on sensitive components of the vertebral column.

It is logical to assume that strong low-back muscles may help prevent low-back problems. Strong low-back muscles provide better musculoskeletal function, support, control, and shock absorption, reducing the risk of low-back injury and structural degeneration.

Morrow (1997) studied low-back pain in more than 3,000 men and women. Those individuals who participated in general strength training activities were about 10% less likely to experience low-back problems than those who did not perform strength exercises.

Although low-back pain is a complex medical problem, an appropriate program of low-back strengthening exercise may be an effective approach for decreasing or preventing low-back discomfort due to weak trunk extensor muscles. It is also likely that a strong midsection musculature (rectus abdominis, external obliques, internal obliques) may help protect low-back structures from physical stress and further reduce the risk of injury.

Arthritis

People who suffer from arthritis often avoid strength training. Yet the few studies completed in this area (Marks 1993; Quirk, Newman, and Newman 1985) indicate that stronger muscles may improve joint function and reduce arthritic discomfort. Although the exact mechanisms by which strength exercise provides relief are not understood, recent research at Tufts University concludes that strength training eases the pain of osteoarthritis and rheumatoid arthritis (Tufts 1994).

At the very least, arthritics who strength train should benefit from a stronger musculoskeletal system and greater joint functional capacity.

Osteoporosis

Osteoporosis is a degenerative disease of the skeletal system characterized by gradual loss of bone proteins and minerals. Because bone condition essentially parallels muscle condition, weak muscles are associated with weak bones and strong muscles with strong bones: the same activities that build myoproteins in our muscles also enhance the protein and mineral content in our bones. Although genetics, hormones, nutrition, and other factors affect bone remodeling and influence the course of osteoporosis, strength training is an excellent way to develop and maintain strong and functional musculoskeletal systems that resist deterioration and osteoporosis (Bell, Godsen, and Henry 1988; Colletti et al. 1989; Ryan et al. 1994; Snow-Harter et al. 1992). Research with older men (Menkes et al. 1993) and postmenopausal women (Nelson et al. 1994) indicate that bone loss can be changed to bone gain through regular and progressive strength training.

The study by Menkes et al. (1993) showed significant increases in bone mineral density at the neck of the femur. This is an important finding because the femoral neck is a common area for fractures in older individuals.

Nelson and her colleagues completed the classic study on strength training and osteoporosis at Tufts University in 1994, with 39 postmenopausal women (ages 50 to 70 years) engaging in a full year of regular strength workouts. The program comprised five machine exercises (hip extension, knee extension, lat pulldown, back extension, abdominal flexion) performed for three sets of eight repetitions, two days per week. The women who performed strength training increased their lumbar spine and femoral neck bone mineral density by 1%. The women who did not do strength exercise experienced a 2% decrease in lumbar spine and femoral neck bone mineral density. The nonexercising group lost over a pound of muscle, whereas the strength-trained women added almost 3 pounds of muscle.

Another 12-month study of menopausal women clearly demonstrated the importance of strength training for increasing bone mineral density (Notelovitz et al. 1991). Subjects who combined strength training and estrogen therapy increased total bone mineral density by 2.1%, whereas those who received only estrogen therapy experienced no change in bone mineral density. Taunton (1997) replicated the results of Notelovitz's (1991) work in a study showing that strength training resulted in an increase in bone mineral density of the lumbar spine and a trend toward improved hip bone mineral density in 65- to 75-year-old women.

These studies provide convincing evidence that strength training can produce positive changes in bone mineral density—which can, in turn, provide some degree of protection from osteoporosis.

Glucose Utilization

Inability of body cells to utilize glucose effectively is a metabolic disorder that may lead to diabetes mellitus. Exercise promotes glucose utilization, and most diabetics find regular exercise useful for maintaining consistent glucose levels. Although aerobic exercise has traditionally been recommended for enhancing glucose utilization (Council on Exercise of The American Diabetes Association 1990), research suggests that strength training may be equally effective (Durak, Jovanovis-Peterson, and Peterson 1990; Miller et al. 1984).

Craig, Everhart, and Brown (1989) showed that 12 weeks of strength training significantly improved insulin response/glucose utilization in both younger (mean age 23 years) and older (mean age 63 years) men. Hurley (1994) reported 23% greater glucose utilization in older men after four months of strength workouts. Eriksson et al. (1997) found that an 11-station circuit weight training program (one set of each exercise, twice a week, for three months) significantly improved glycemic control in previously sedentary seniors with type II diabetes.

Diabetics may benefit from strength training in many ways. First, strength training may reverse muscle myopathy, a problem associated with poor glucose utilization and a predisposing factor for adult onset diabetes (Durak 1989). Second, strength training may preserve lean body mass in people who follow low-calorie diets to reduce body fat (Ballor et al. 1988). Third, trained muscles have higher glucose uptake and lower insulin resistance than untrained muscles (Lohmann and Liebold 1978).

Because poor glucose metabolism is a predisposing factor in type II diabetes, strength training's positive effect on glucose uptake may help prevent this prevalent disease in older adults.

Gastrointestinal Transit

Gastrointestinal transit refers to the time required for food to move through the digestive system. Slow gastrointestinal transit speed appears to be associated with increased risk for colon cancer (Hurley 1994). Aerobic activity such as running has been shown to speed up gastrointestinal transit (Cordain, Latin, and Behnke 1986), perhaps as a result of muscular contractions that affect the system components.

More recently, researchers at the University of Maryland found that strength training produced faster gastrointestinal transit in middle-aged and older men (Koffler et al. 1992). The subjects' average gastrointestinal transit time decreased 56% after just three months of strength training. The researchers concluded that strength training may be an effective way to address age-related gastrointestinal motility disorders, as well as to reduce the risk of colon cancer.

Blood Pressure

Exercise increases demands on the cardiovascular system, resulting in both higher heart rate and higher systolic blood pressure. Although continuous tension exercise (such as isometric muscle contractions) can increase blood pressure to dangerous levels, this does not seem to occur with standard strength training. A study of upper body strength exercise showed a temporary systolic blood pressure increase of 34% (Westcott and Howes 1983), and a study of lower body strength exercise revealed a 50% elevation (Westcott 1986). These responses are well within normal limits, and compare favorably to systolic blood pressure increases during aerobic exercise (Westcott 1986).

Although strength training produces temporary elevations in blood pressure during the activity session, it does not result in higher resting blood pressure levels following a program of strength training (Hurley 1994). Comparative studies show that strength training and aerobic exercise are equally effective in reducing resting blood pressure (Blumenthal, Siegel and Appelbaum 1991; Smutok et al. 1993).

In several studies, regular strength training has actually led to a decrease in resting blood pressure (systolic, diastolic, or both). Research by Wilmore et al. (1976) noted reductions in diastolic blood pressure following 10 weeks of circuit weight training; Harris and Holly (1987) observed lower diastolic readings after nine weeks of circuit weight training; and Hurley et al. (1988) demonstrated decreased diastolic blood pressures after 16 weeks of circuit weight training. Meta-analysis of nine studies on blood pressure response to weight training revealed average reductions of about 3% for resting systolic blood pressure and about 4% for resting diastolic blood pressure (Kelly 1997).

A study of older men and women (mean age 57 years) by Westcott, Dolan, and Cavicchi (1996) showed significant reduction in systolic blood pressure following eight weeks of circuit weight training. Other strength training studies (Blumenthal, Siegel and Appelbaum 1991; Katz and Wilson 1992) have revealed reductions in both systolic and diastolic blood pressures, but the changes did not differ significantly from the non-exercising control groups.

Contrary to popular misconceptions, sensible strength training does not appear to have detrimental effects on blood pressure; and several studies have shown that circuit weight training programs may significantly reduce resting blood pressure levels.

Blood Lipids

Blood lipid profiles appear to be important predictors of cardiovascular disease. Unfortunately, many older adults have levels of total cholesterol, LDL (bad) cholesterol, and triglycerides that are higher than desirable, and levels of HDL (good) cholesterol that are lower than desirable. Although genetics is a major factor in this area, research indicates that diet and exercise may have some influence on blood lipid profiles.

Aerobic exercise and strength training appear to have similar effects on blood lipids (Blessing, Stone, and Byrd 1987; Johnson et al. 1982; Smutok et al. 1993). Goldberg et al. (1984), Stone et al. (1982), Ulrich, Reid, and Yeater (1987), and Boyden et al. (1993) observed improved blood lipid profiles following various programs of strength training.

Perhaps the best known study on this topic was conducted by Hurley et al. in 1988. Their subjects (40- to 55-year-old men) significantly decreased LDL cholesterol and significantly increased HDL cholesterol after 16 weeks of circuit weight training. However, other studies conducted by Hurley and his associates did not demonstrate significant improvements in blood lipid levels (Kokkinos et al. 1988; Kokkinos et al. 1991; Smutok et al. 1993).

Because the studies on strength training's effectiveness for improving blood lipid profiles are not conclusive, more research is warranted. We at least can be confident in saying that regular strength exercise does not adversely affect blood lipid profiles, and *may* produce desirable changes in LDL and HDL cholesterol levels.

Postcoronary Performance

Coronary artery disease is the leading medical problem in the United States, and is particularly prevalent among older adults. Fortunately, treatment of coronary artery disease has progressed to the point where many heart attack survivors and postbypass patients lead relatively normal lives. Although usually encouraged to walk, patients with cardiovascular problems have traditionally been advised against resistance exercise—an unfortunate situation, since recovering individuals experience reduced physical activity and muscle atrophy during their rehabilitation period. They, like everyone else, are dependent upon their muscular fitness to perform physical tasks and daily activities. Sensible strength training appears to be a safe and effective means for improving muscular fitness and physical performance in postcoronary patients. It is also useful for maintaining a desirable bodyweight and positive self-concept, both of which are important to many individuals who have experienced coronary problems.

A three-year study at Johns Hopkins University (Stewart, Mason, and Kelemen 1988) showed that circuit strength training increased muscular strength and self-confidence in cardiac patients. Another study at the same institution (Kelemen et al. 1986) demonstrated significant improvements in muscle strength and aerobic endurance in cardiac patients between 35 and 70 years of age.

Several studies have shown that sensible strength training is a safe and productive activity for most postcoronary patients (Butler, Beierwaltes, and Rogers 1987; Faigenbaum et al. 1990; Ghilarducci, Holly, and Amsterdam 1989; Haennel, Quinney, and Kappagoda 1991; Vander et al. 1986). The American College of Sports Medicine (1991) has suggested that asymptomatic cardiac patients begin low-level resistance exercise as soon as seven to eight weeks after their event; and the American Association of Cardiovascular and Pulmonary Rehabilitation (1995) has developed a comprehensive set of strength training recommendations for postcoronary individuals.

Stronger musculoskeletal systems render routine and unplanned activities less stressful on the cardiovascular system, thereby reducing cardiac risk. Of course, medical approval is essential prior to placing postcoronary patients on a strength training program.

Self-Confidence and Depression

Self-confidence includes many factors that combine to give a perspective on one's ability to function at home, at work, in recreational activities, or at social events. Westcott (1995) attempted to ascertain self-confidence levels of 48 middle-aged and older adults before and after an eight-week program of strength and endurance exercise. All of the participants rated their self-confidence on an anonymous, written questionnaire using a five-point scale (5 = high; 1 = low). Prior to the exercise program the mean self-confidence level was 3.3; after eight weeks of training the mean level of self-confidence was 3.8. Although statistical analyses were not performed, these results suggest that the exercise program was a positive experience for the participants with respect to self-confidence.

A recent study conducted at Harvard Medical School (Singh, Clements, and Fiatarone 1997) suggests that older adults who suffer from depression may benefit from strength training. The 32 subjects (age range 60 to 84 years) met the diagnostic criteria for mild to moderate depression and were assigned to either a strength training program or a lecture/discussion series on health-related topics. After 10 weeks, 82% of the strength exercisers no longer met the depression criteria, compared to 40% of the health class participants.

Although more research is needed in these areas, it would appear that strength training may be beneficial for enhancing self-confidence and counteracting depression in older adults.

Summary of Strength Training Benefits

Research indicates that older adults may experience many health-related benefits from a sensible program of strength exercise that is performed at a relatively high-effort level. Some of the possible benefits include the following:

- *Better body composition,* with up to 4 pounds more lean weight and 4 pounds less fat weight after two months of regular strength training.

- *Increased metabolic rate,* with up to 7% higher resting metabolism and up to 15% greater daily calorie requirements after three months of regular strength exercise.

- *Decreased low back discomfort,* with approximately 80% of patients reporting less or no pain after about three months of specific low-back strengthening exercise.

- *Reduced arthritic pain,* as indicated by subjective ratings of symptoms in strength-trained adults who have arthritis.

- *Increased bone mineral density* that may prevent age-related bone loss and offer protection against osteoporosis.

- *Enhanced glucose utilization* that may reduce the risk of type II diabetes.

- *Faster gastrointestinal transit* that may reduce the risk of colon cancer and other motility disorders of the gastrointestinal system.

- *Reduced resting blood pressure,* including lower diastolic readings and lower systolic readings.

- *Improved blood lipid profiles,* including lower levels of LDL cholesterol and higher levels of HDL cholesterol.

- *Improved postcoronary performance* resulting from higher muscular functional capacity and lower cardiovascular stress from routine and unplanned physical activity.

- *Enhanced self-confidence,* as reported by previously sedentary men and women following two months of regular strength training.

- *Relieved depression* in older adults clinically diagnosed with mild to moderate depression.

chapter two

Training Principles to Use With Seniors

Muscle strength can be developed by almost any training program that progressively increases the exercise resistance. Unfortunately, some popular strength training protocols carry a high risk of injury while others provide a low rate of improvement. A well-designed strength training program for older adults should minimize injury potential and maximize muscle responsiveness. It also should be relatively time-efficient and simple to perform. Senior strength trainers may work at relatively high-effort levels (Fiatarone et al. 1990; Frontera et al. 1988; Nelson et al. 1994), but should not push so hard that their muscles are sore on the days between workouts (Miles et al. 1997).

In 1990, the American College of Sports Medicine (ACSM) released general guidelines for safely achieving higher levels of muscle fitness through strength training. According to the ACSM, a basic program of strength training should include at least one set of 8 to 12 repetitions of 8 to 10 exercises for the major muscle groups, performed at least two days a week.

This chapter presents more detailed information on designing effective strength training programs for older adults. We address the key program components of

- training frequency
- training sets
- exercise resistance
- exercise repetitions

- training progression, and
- exercise selection.

Training Frequency

Properly performed strength training exercises progressively stress the prime mover muscles and produce some degree of *tissue microtrauma*. Following each exercise session, the stressed tissues undergo repair and building processes that result in larger and stronger muscles. These beneficial physiological adaptations typically require 48 to 96 hours to occur, and it is during this time frame that the next strength workout should be undertaken for best training results. Thus, strength development is enhanced by training again two to four days after the last workout. Conversely, training more frequently prevents the muscles from developing to their full potential, and training less frequently passes over the optimum period for progressively building greater strength.

Individual differences will vary the amount of recovery time needed to achieve maximum muscle-building benefit. You must therefore monitor your clients' improvement carefully to determine the most productive training frequency for each person.

> **Tissue Microtrauma:** *Microscopic tears in muscle and connective tissue that require about 48 to 96 hours recovery time for remodeling and building processes to be completed.*

Because the only way to determine an exerciser's most productive training frequency is through trial and error, it is important to maintain a detailed record of each client's training sessions. When the muscle recovery and building period between workouts is appropriate, you should consistently and progressively increase your client's exercise repetitions and/or weightloads.

Although most strength training textbooks recommend three strength training sessions per week (Baechle and Groves 1998; Fleck and Kraemer 1997; Westcott 1995), some research indicates that two strength workouts per week may be as effective (Braith et al. 1989; DeMichele et al. 1997). Specifically, twice-a-week strength training appears to be highly productive for men and women over the age of 50 (Stadler, Stubbs, and Vukovich 1997; Westcott and Guy 1996).

In 1989, Braith et al. found that two exercise sessions per week produced 75% as much strength gains as three training sessions. However, a 1997 study from the same university (DeMichele et al. 1997) showed equal strength development from two or three weight training workouts per week. Both the

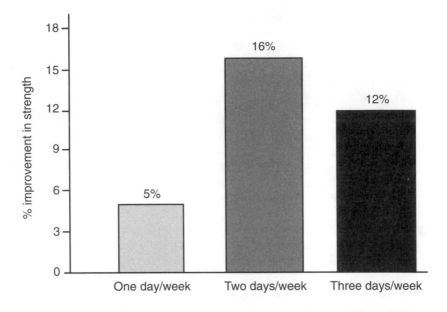

Figure 2.1   Strength gains after 12 weeks of training one, two, or three days per week (DeMichele et al. 1997).

two- and three-day trainees showed similar strength gains (figure 2.1), but the subjects who trained only once a week did not make significant strength changes.

Older men and women who trained two or three times per week showed similar improvements in muscle strength (Stadler, Stubbs, and Vucovich 1997). Westcott and Guy (1996) compared body composition changes for 1,132 younger, middle-aged, and older adults who performed two or three strength training sessions per week. In all age categories (21-40 years, 41-60 years, 61-80 years), the twice-a-week trainees experienced about 90% as much muscle gain and fat loss as those who did three workouts per week.

Summary—Studies On Training Frequency

Braith et al. 1989: 2 days 75% as effective as 3 days for strength development.

Westcott and Guy 1996: 2 days 90% as effective as 3 days for muscle development.

DeMichele et al. 1997: 2 days as effective as 3 days for strength development.

Stadler, Stubbs, and Vucovich 1997: 2 days as effective as 3 days for strength development.

General Guideline: The general guideline for training frequency is two or three exercise sessions per week on nonconsecutive days.

Specific Guideline: We recommend spacing strength workouts as evenly as possible. For example, Mondays, Wednesdays, and Fridays for three-day trainees, or Mondays and Thursdays for two-day trainees.

Training consistency is as important as frequency. Obviously, missing scheduled training sessions is unproductive due to the lack of a strength-building stimulus. Yet working the same muscles two days in succession can be counterproductive due to insufficient time for muscle recovery and remodeling. We suggest that older adults make it a high priority—even if some lifestyle changes are required—to schedule regular workouts that foster progressive strength development.

Training Sets

According to the 1990 training guidelines of the American College of Sports Medicine, one or more sets of resistance exercise are recommended for developing muscle strength. Although some trainers prefer multiple-set training programs, one set is the minimum requirement for stimulating strength gains; and because single-set strength training provides a user-friendly and time-efficient approach to muscle fitness, it is a suggested starting point for most older adults.

Although competitive weightlifters and bodybuilders perform several sets of each exercise, high-volume strength training (large numbers of sets and repetitions) may not be necessary for improving muscle fitness in average adults. In fact, several studies have demonstrated similar results from single-set and multiple-set strength training, at least for the first four months of exercise.

A 14-week study by Starkey et al. (1996) compared lower body strength gains for 38 untrained adults who completed one or three sets of exercise. Both exercise groups attained similar increases in lower body strength, as indicated by their performance improvement in knee extension and knee flexion exercises.

Kraemer (Kraemer, Purvis, and Westcott 1996) reported a nine-month study with college athletes who performed either single-set or multiple-set strength training. Both groups experienced similar strength improvement over the first four months of training, after which the multiple-set exercise program produced better results.

Westcott, Greenberger, and Milius (1989) examined muscle endurance changes in 77 middle-aged men and women who completed one, two, or three sets of exercise over a 10-week training period. All three exercise groups experienced similar increases in upper body muscle endurance, as indicated by their performance improvement in chin-ups and bar-dips.

With respect to muscle development, Westcott and Guy (1996) assessed changes in lean weight for 1,132 men and women following eight weeks of single-set strength training. All three age groups (21-40 years, 41-60 years, 61-80 years) added similar and significant amounts of lean weight, indicating that single-set strength training is an efficient and effective means for building muscle in beginning adult exercisers during the first two months of training.

Summary—Studies on Training Sets

Starkey et al. 1996: 1 or 3 sets equally effective for strength development over 14-week training period.

Kraemer, Purvis, and Westcott 1996: single or multiple sets equally effective for strength development over 16-week training period with multiple sets more productive than single sets for strength development after 16 weeks of training.

Westcott, Greenberger, and Milius 1989: 1, 2, or 3 sets equally effective for muscle endurance development over 10-week training period.

Westcott and Guy 1996: single set training effective for muscle development in beginning adult and senior exercisers.

General Guideline: The general guideline for training sets is one set of each exercise for new participants. More advanced trainees may perform two or three sets of each exercise if they have the desire and ability to complete higher volume workouts.

Specific Guideline: We suggest that when performing two or more sets of the same exercise, clients should rest approximately two minutes between sets. This provides the time needed to replenish about 95% of the energy stores used during the previous exercise set. Taking shorter rest periods may reduce the number of repetitions completed on subsequent sets of an exercise.

One method for performing multiple sets is to do the same number of repetitions with the same weightload for each set of a given exercise. For example, a client may complete three sets of 10 leg presses using 100 pounds for each set.

Another approach to multiple-set training is to do the same number of repetitions with progressively heavier weightloads for each set of a given exercise. For example, the same client may perform a set of 10 leg presses with 60 pounds, a set of 10 leg presses with 80 pounds, and a set of 10 leg presses with 100 pounds. There is some evidence (Faigenbaum et al. 1993; Faigenbaum et al. 1996) that, for beginning participants, three exercise sets with progressively heavier weightloads may have greater effect than three sets with the same resistance.

In summary, older adults are well advised to start strength training with one set of exercise for all of the major muscle groups. As training continues and their muscle fitness improves, you may want to have your clients perform additional sets. Multiple sets of a given exercise may be performed with the same resistance or with progressively heavier weightloads. When doing multiple sets of an exercise, clients should rest approximately two minutes between sets to allow intracellular energy stores to be replenished.

Exercise Resistance

The basic premise of strength training is to use weightloads that make muscles work harder than they are accustomed to working. This process has traditionally been called *overload*, and indicates training with progressively heavier weightloads to stimulate further strength development. For example, an exerciser currently training with 50-pound arm curls could experience an overload effect by increasing the weightload to 52.5 pounds.

The overload principle may be applied to any exercise resistance, but most authorities advise training loads that equal between 60 and 90% of maximum resistance (Baechle and Earle 1995). Maximum resistance represents the heaviest weightload that can be lifted one time and is referred to as the 1 RM. Exercise resistance and training repetitions are inversely related: lower weightloads permit more repetitions, and higher weightloads require fewer repetitions. For example, a client may complete 16 repetitions with 60% of maximum resistance, but only four repetitions with 90% of maximum resistance. Using 60% of maximum resistance has both a lower strength-building stimulus and a lower risk of injury; 90% of maximum resistance provides a higher strength-building stimulus, but a higher risk of injury.

We recommend that beginners train with about 70 to 80% of maximum resistance. Workloads in this range provide both high strength-building stimulus and low risk of injury. Research studies with subjects in their 60s, 70s, 80s, and 90s have shown excellent results with training loads between 70 to 80% of maximum resistance, which corresponds to about 8-12 repetitions for most exercises. Selected studies are summarized below.

Summary—Studies on Exercise Resistance

Frontera et al. 1988: Men in their 60s and 70s experienced significant increases in muscle mass and strength after 12 weeks of training with 80% of maximum resistance.

Fiatarone et al. 1990: Men and women in their 90s experienced significant increases in muscle mass and strength after eight weeks of training with 80% of maximum resistance.

Nelson et al. 1994: Women in their 50s and 60s experienced significant increases in muscle mass and strength after 50 weeks of training with 80% of maximum resistance.

Westcott and Guy 1996: Men and women in their 50s, 60s, 70s, and 80s experienced significant increases in muscle mass and strength after eight weeks of training with 70 to 80% of maximum resistance.

General Guideline: The general guideline for training resistance is weightloads between 70 to 80% of maximum resistance.

Specific Guidelines: Training with weightloads between 60 to 70% of maximum resistance may result in a slightly lower rate of strength development and a slightly lower risk of injury.

Training with weightloads between 80 to 90% of maximum resistance may result in a slightly higher rate of strength development and a slightly higher risk of injury.

Years of empirical evidence and many research studies support training with exercise resistance between 70 to 80% of maximum. We therefore suggest that older adults typically train with about 70 to 80% of their maximum resistance. Lower weightloads (60 to 70% of maximum) may be advisable during the initial training period; higher weightloads (80 to 90% of maximum) may be preferred as participants become more advanced. Periodically training with different percentages of maximum resistance provides a change of pace that may have both physiological and psychological benefits.

Exercise Repetitions

As noted in the previous section, there is an inverse relationship between the resistance used and the number of repetitions that can be completed. Most adults can complete about 8-12 repetitions with 75% of their maximum resistance (Westcott 1995). As shown in figure 2.2, only a small percentage of subjects performed fewer than eight repetitions (power athletes) or more than 12 repetitions (endurance athletes) when tested with 75% of their maximum resistance in a chest exercise. The mean number of repetitions completed in this study was 10, indicating that the 10-repetition weightload is about 75% of maximum resistance.

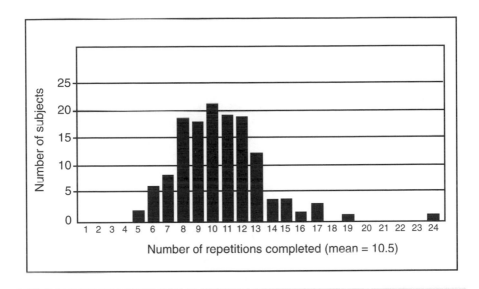

Figure 2.2 Distribution of repetitions completed with 75% of maximum weightload (N = 141).

For practical purposes it is not necessary to find an individual's maximum resistance to determine the 75% weightload. In most cases, if a weightload can be performed for 10 repetitions using correct form it will be approximately 75% of one's maximum resistance, and is an appropriate training load. Because finding the one-repetition maximum weightload for a previously sedentary senior poses an injury risk, it is not a recommended procedure.

The subjects in the aforementioned study (Westcott 1995) performed each exercise repetition in about six seconds, completing 8-12 repetitions in approximately 50 to 70 seconds. This represents a *high-effort set* of *anaerobic exercise*, which is the essential stimulus for strength development.

> **High-Effort Set:** *A challenging series of repetitions that terminates when the weightload cannot be lifted with proper form.*

> **Anaerobic Exercise:** *Demanding physical activity that exceeds the energy production capacity of the oxygen system and cannot be performed for more than about 90 seconds at a time.*

Just as there is a range of productive exercise resistances, there is a corresponding range of effective training repetitions. Figure 2.3 illustrates a continuum of resistance and repetitions relationships for the recommended strength training protocols.

> **General Guideline:** *The general guideline for training repetitions is 8-12 repetitions per set, performed with proper technique to the point of muscle fatigue. This is typically accomplished with weightloads between 70 to 80% of maximum.*

> **Specific Guidelines:** *Training with more than 12 repetitions per set may result in a slightly lower rate of strength development, but carries a slightly lower risk of injury.*
>
> *Training with fewer than eight repetitions per set may result in a slightly higher rate of strength development, but carries a slightly higher risk of injury.*

Older adult strength training studies presented in the previous section utilized similar training procedures, namely 8-12 repetitions per set with 70 to 80% of maximum resistance. Higher repetitions (more than 12 reps) with lower weightloads may be advisable during the initial training period, when older adults are learning proper exercise technique. Lower repetitions (fewer than 8 reps) may be preferred as clients become stronger and require more demanding training protocols.

As presented in chapter 6 (pages 142 and 144), higher repetitions with lighter weightloads emphasize muscle endurance development, whereas fewer repetitions with heavier weightloads emphasize muscle strength development.

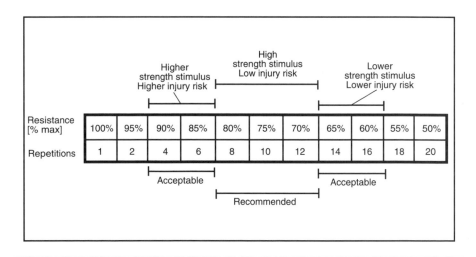

Figure 2.3   Resistance and repetitions relationships for the recommended strength training protocols.

Training Progression

As training continues and the muscles become stronger, more repetitions can be completed with a given weightload. Increasing the number of repetitions is a logical approach to training progression and is a productive procedure up to a point. For best results, however, individuals should complete each exercise set within the time frame of the anaerobic energy system—typically requiring 8-12 repetitions, or about 50 to 70 seconds of continuous training effort.

Based on this standard training range of 8-12 repetitions, your clients should slightly raise their exercise weightloads whenever they complete 12 repetitions with proper form on two consecutive workouts. Although there are no studies on specific load increments, our observations suggest that resistance increases of 5% or less provide safe and productive training progression.

General Guideline: The general guideline for training progression is to increase the exercise weightload by 5% or less whenever 12 repetitions are completed with correct form in two consecutive workouts.

Specific Guideline: For practical purposes, we recommend 2.5-pound resistance increments, as this represents the minimum weightload increase for dumbbells, barbells, and most weightstack machines.

First increasing the number of repetitions, and then increasing the weightload, is a protocol known as a *double progressive program*—a conservative training approach that reduces risks of overtraining injuries.

Double Progressive Program: Systematically increasing the training demands by first adding more repetitions, then adding more resistance.

You can apply the double progressive program to other training protocols. For example, trainees performing 12 to 16 repetitions per set should add 2.5 pounds upon completing 16 repetitions in two successive training sessions.

Exercise Selection and Sequence

Although a sound strength training program should address all of the major muscle groups (ACSM 1990), many people take a "preferred exercise" approach—they select certain exercises that are more popular, more convenient, or more satisfying to perform. For example, many strength training enthusiasts emphasize the bench press, which is an excellent exercise for the pectoralis major, anterior deltoid, and triceps muscles. However, if equal attention is not given to the *opposing muscles* (latissimus dorsi, teres major, posterior deltoid, and biceps), *muscle imbalance* is likely to develop around the shoulder joint due to a relatively strong chest musculature and a relatively weak upper back musculature. Such imbalances may lead to poor posture and musculoskeletal injuries.

> **Opposing Muscles:** *Muscles that produce the opposite joint movements of the prime mover muscles.*

> **Muscle Imbalance:** *The condition in which one muscle is disproportionately stronger than its opposing muscle.*

To facilitate balanced muscle development, we recommend pairing exercises for opposing muscle groups. For example, if the first exercise in a machine strength training session is the leg extension for the quadriceps muscles, the second exercise is the leg curl for the hamstrings muscles. A workout with free weights may start with squats for the same muscles, as this exercise works both the quadriceps and the hamstrings simultaneously.

The next group of exercises should address the torso muscles, including the pectoralis major, latissimus dorsi, and deltoid groups. Sample exercises include machine chest crossovers and dumbbell flys for the pectoralis major; machine pullovers and dumbbell bent rows for the latissimus dorsi; and both machine and dumbbell lateral raises for the deltoids.

Next in the training sequence are the biceps and triceps, which may be worked effectively with machine or dumbbell curls and machine or dumbbell extensions.

The final muscles worked in the suggested training sequence are the midsection and neck groups. Because these muscles serve as stabilizers in most exercises, it is best not to fatigue them until the end of the workout. Recommended midsection exercises include the low-back machine and abdominal machine, as well as trunk extensions and trunk curls with bodyweight resistance. The neck muscles may be exercised safely and effectively on the neck machine.

In addition to using the basic exercises, older adults may benefit by strengthening the adductor and abductor muscles of the hip, the oblique muscles that surround the midsection, the calf muscles, and the forearm muscles. We recommend including exercises for these muscle groups in the overall training program on a regular basis if possible. Table 2.1 presents sample machine and free-weight exercises for all major muscle groups, and lists the pages on which these exercises are illustrated and described in chapter 4.

Table 2.1

Recommended Performance Sequence of Machine and Free-Weight Exercises

Muscle group	Machine exercise	Free-weight exercise
Quadriceps	Leg extension machine (p. 44)	Dumbbell squat (p. 48)
Hamstrings	Leg curl machine (p. 46)	Dumbbell squat (p. 48)
Hip adductors	Hip adductor machine (p. 54)	– – – – – – – – – – – – –
Hip abductors	Hip abductor machine (p. 56)	– – – – – – – – – – – – –
Gastrocnemius	Standing calf machine (p. 62)	Dumbbell heel raise (p. 58)
Pectoralis major	Chest cross machine (p. 74)	Dumbbell bench press (p. 80)
Latissimus dorsi	Pullover machine (p. 86)	Dumbbell one-arm row (p. 88)
Deltoids	Lateral raise machine (p. 98)	Dumbbell press (p. 96)
Biceps	Biceps machine (p. 106)	Dumbbell biceps curl (p. 108)
Triceps	Triceps machine (p. 114)	Dumbbell overhead triceps extension (p. 116)
Low back	Low back machine (p. 64)	Low back extension (p. 66)
Abdominals	Abdominal machine (p. 68)	Trunk curl (p. 70)
Obliques	Rotary torso machine (p. 72)	Twisting trunk curl (p. 160)
Neck extensors	Neck machine (p. 122)	– – – – – – – – – – – – –
Neck flexors	Neck machine (p. 120)	– – – – – – – – – – – – –
Forearms	Forearm machine (p. 124)	Dumbbell biceps curl (p. 108)

You may want to match the exercises with the muscle groups they address, as presented in the muscle illustrations at the beginning of chapter 4.

> *General Guideline:* The general guideline for exercise selection is one exercise for each of the major muscle groups. Exercises should include the quadriceps, hamstrings, pectoralis major, latissimus dorsi, deltoids, biceps, triceps, low back, abdominals, and neck, as well as the hip adductors, hip abductors, obliques, calves, and forearms.

> *Special Guideline:* We recommend pairing exercises for opposing muscle groups, and training larger muscles before smaller muscles.

Although it may be advisable to perform a specific exercise for each major muscle group, time and equipment limitations may make this difficult to accomplish. If this is the case, a smaller number of *multiple-muscle exercises* may

Table 2.2

Sample Abbreviated Machine and Free-Weight Exercise Program

Muscle groups	Machine exercise	Free-weight exercise
Quadriceps, hamstrings	Leg press machine (p. 52)	Dumbbell squat (p. 48)
Pectoralis major, triceps, deltoids	Chest press machine (p. 78)	Bench press (p. 80)
Latissimus dorsi, biceps, deltoids	Compound row machine (p. 90)	Dumbbell one-arm row (p. 88)
Obliques, abdominals	Rotary torso machine (p. 72)	Twisting trunk curl (p. 160)

provide a similar conditioning effect. Table 2.2 presents an abbreviated strength training program that addresses most of the major muscle groups with just four exercises. The pages on which these exercises are illustrated and described are also listed in table 2.2. Whether your clients perform many or few exercises, they should train the major muscle groups in a comprehensive manner that increases overall strength and function.

Multiple-Muscle Exercises: Exercises that use two or more major muscle groups simultaneously to perform the required movement pattern.

Summary of Strength Training Guidelines for Older Adults

The following guidelines should provide a sensible framework for designing safe and successful strength training programs for older adults.

Training Frequency

The general guideline for training frequency is two or three exercise sessions per week on nonconsecutive days. Research indicates that two workouts per week produce 88% of the gain in muscle mass and strength as three workouts per week.

Training Sets

The general guideline for training sets is one set of each exercise for new participants. More advanced trainees may perform two or three sets of each exercise. Studies show that single-set training is as effective as multiple-set protocols for the first four months of strength exercise.

Exercise Resistance

The general guideline for training resistance emphasizes weightloads between 70 to 80% of maximum resistance. Research reveals that weightloads in this training range are safe and effective for increasing muscle mass and strength in older adults.

Exercise Repetitions

The general guideline for repetitions is 8-12 reps per set, performed with proper technique to the point of muscle fatigue. Studies show that 8-12 repetitions can typically be completed with weightloads between 70 to 80% of maximum resistance.

Training Progression

The general guideline for training progression is to increase the exercise resistance by 5% or less whenever 12 repetitions can be completed with correct form in two successive workouts. This represents a double progressive training program, first adding more repetitions and then adding more resistance.

Exercise Selection

The general guideline for exercise selection is one exercise for each of the major muscle groups. We recommend training larger muscles before training smaller muscles, and working opposing muscle groups in pairs. Chapters 5 and 6 present exercise arrangements.

chapter three

Teaching Strategies and Training Procedures

Teaching strength training concepts and techniques to older adults requires both a thorough knowledge of correct exercise movements and a strong sensitivity to the uniqueness of this group of clients. Successful instruction also involves a well-planned and sequential presentation of the exercise techniques, as well as an understanding of strength training procedures that will make your teaching approaches safe and effective. Just as important as educating older adults about strength exercise is motivating them to begin and continue a personal program of strength training.

Motivating older adults to train consistently and correctly can be a challenging task. The newness of the activity, the fear of injury, the potential embarrassment of appearing weak or uncoordinated, the concern of giving good effort without getting noticeable results, as well as various misconceptions and distractions—all these factors make it more difficult for older adults than for younger adults to master strength training skills.

Successful instructors do not merely teach how to perform exercise—they actually shape older adults' attitudes towards strength training. For best results, both the process and the product of sensible strength training must be positive experiences. The following teaching strategies have proven effective for motivating mature adults to do strength training with a high level of cooperation and satisfaction.

Teaching Strategies

Although some older adults may be enthusiastic about exercise, most require extrinsic motivation to maintain their interest and adherence, especially during the first few weeks of training.

The Four Focus Words

You should say four key words to each participant during every exercise session: *Hello, Goodbye, Thank You,* and the *Individual's Name.* Of course, *Hello* and *Goodbye* need be used only once, when the client arrives and departs. *Thank you* may be used as often as appropriate, and the *Individual's Name* should be spoken frequently. These are the *Four Focus Words* that make new exercisers feel noticed, valued, and appreciated as a participant in the strength training program.

> ***Four Focus Words:*** *Use with each participant during every class.*
>
> - *Hello!*
> - *Thank You!*
> - *Goodbye!*
> - *Individual's Name*

The Ten Teaching Statements

While the four focus words represent common courtesy, there are several suggested dialogues that should be standard strategy for older adults, especially during the learning stages of strength training. We refer to these as the *Ten Teaching Statements.* These instructional interactions have proven helpful in large-scale senior strength training programs (Westcott 1995a), and should facilitate positive and productive exercise experiences for new participants.

1. ***Understandable Performance Objectives.*** The first and perhaps most important instructional step is to clearly communicate the client's main performance objective for the class session. That is, tell the exerciser specifically what you want him or her to accomplish during the workout. This provides training direction and enables the client to focus on the major task rather than less substantive details.

2. ***Concise Instruction with Precise Demonstration.*** Once you have presented the performance objective, provide simple instructions on how to accomplish it: tell the client exactly what he or she should do. Because *showing* is typically more effective than *telling*, the next instructional step is modeling the desired exercise actions. The demonstration phase should be deliberate rather than rushed, and repeated as many times as necessary. Introduce

additional exercises only after your clients' exercise form and breathing patterns are flawless. Always point out key aspects of proper technique during the demonstration.

3. *Attentive Supervision.* Never assume that people understand exactly how to do what you have just demonstrated, or are able to do so without coaching. Stay beside your client during their first attempts to replicate your exercise movement patterns. Many older individuals lack confidence in their physical ability, while others have limited neuromuscular coordination. In either case, by being watchful you can boost confidence and reduce the fear of making a mistake. Attentive supervision is a powerful motivator for most new exercisers.

4. *Appropriate Assistance.* To assure safe and successful exercise performance, you may need to provide some form of manual assistance for many older adults. This may include assisting clients onto a machine, helping them fasten a seat belt, handing them free weights, guiding them through an exercise movement, stabilizing their posture, or making minor adjustments to body part positions. Whereas younger exercisers may be less receptive to manual assistance, most older adults appreciate a helping hand as they attempt to master new strength exercises.

5. *One Task at a Time.* Presenting several simultaneous or sequential performance tasks may be confusing or even overwhelming to older adults. Give only one instructional request at a time. Providing a single directive increases the probability that your client will successfully complete each task and feel more physically competent and mentally confident.

6. *Gradual Progression.* While the essence of strength training is progression, it is necessary to progress relatively slowly with older adults. Never introduce a follow-up task until the first task has been performed properly, and always present simple actions before more complex actions. For older individuals, approach strength training as a series of hurdles, with the first hurdle very low and each successive hurdle just a little bit higher.

7. *Positive Reinforcement.* Most older exercisers experience some degree of uncertainty over the effectiveness of their efforts. Positive reinforcement in the form of encouraging comments, personal compliments, or pats on the shoulder are simple ways to support a person's training progress. Of course, positive reinforcement must be merited and sincere to be meaningful.

8. *Specific Feedback.* Positive reinforcement is more effective when coupled with specific feedback that provides useful information about the exercise performance. Giving a reason for your positive comment makes it more valuable as an educational and motivational tool. Saying "Good job, Jim," may be emotionally reinforcing; but saying "Good job, Jim—you performed all 10 leg curls through a full range of movement" is more informative and more powerful. First, it shows Jim that you were actually observing his exercise form;

second, it increases the likelihood that Jim will again use full movement range the next time he performs leg curls.

9. *Careful Questioning.* Older adults are usually communicative, but they may not volunteer information that could be useful for fine-tuning their training program. Ask relevant questions to learn how they are responding to the exercise experience. Whenever possible, phrase your questions in a manner that promotes thoughtful answers rather than "yes" or "no" responses.

10. *Pre- and Postexercise Dialogue.* Try to sandwich each exercise session between an arriving and departing dialogue. Take a couple of minutes before and after each workout to share some of the participant's perspectives. Pre- and post-training conversations provide opportunities for encouragement and reinforcement, as well as time to become better acquainted with your client.

Table 3.1 presents more detailed information on teaching strategies, with sample instructional statements and specific task descriptions. Use these simple dialogues only as examples for how the 10 suggested client interactions can be implemented.

An Instruction Model

Here is a suggested pattern for presenting strength exercises:

1. Demonstrate how the exercise is performed.
2. Explain each movement phase and the proper breathing pattern.
3. Demonstrate the exercise again with emphasis on proper breathing.
4. Have the client perform the exercise as you breathe with him or her.
5. Provide positive reinforcement for correct technique, with specific feedback and appropriate suggestions for improved performance.

Training Procedures

Your client's most critical concern is how to perform exercises properly. In addition to the unique performance pattern of each exercise, three key components of desirable training technique are full movement range, controlled movement speed, and continuous breathing. Add to this the assignment of appropriate weightloads and purposeful warm-up and cooldown phases, and older adults should experience safe and successful strength training workouts.

Movement Range

Exercising through the full range of joint movement is important for two reasons. Full-range strength training enhances joint flexibility (Westcott

Table 3.1

Sample Instructional Statements
for Implementing Desired Teaching Strategies

General teaching strategy	Sample instructional statement	Specific task description
1. Understandable performance objective	This is what I would like for you to accomplish today.	Your primary task is to exhale during the lifting phase of every repetition.
2. Concise instruction with precise demonstration	This is how I would like for you to breathe when you lift the weightstack.	Watch me breathe out through my mouth during every lifting action.
3. Attentive supervision	I will watch you as you perform the leg extension exercise.	Let me hear you exhale every time you lift the weightstack.
4. Appropriate assistance	I will exhale loud enough for you to hear me during each of your lifting repetitions.	Try to exhale when you hear me breathing out.
5. One task at a time	Remember, all I want you to do is exhale when you lift the weightstack.	Just try to breathe out when you hear me breathe out.
6. Gradual progression	Don't worry about when to inhale. That will be our next task.	If you breathe out when you lift the dumbbell, you should automatically breathe in when you lower the dumbbell.
7. Positive reinforcement	You are doing very well today.	I'm really pleased with your progress.
8. Specific feedback	Your breathing technique is right on target.	You are exhaling evenly throughout every lifting movement.
9. Careful questioning	Do you understand proper breathing for strength exercise?	How does the breathing pattern feel to you?
10. Pre- and postexercise dialogue	Let's talk for a couple minutes about today's exercise experience.	I think you had a great workout, and it looks like you've mastered the breathing technique. Please tell me how you feel about today's training session.

1995b), and full-range exercise movements are necessary to develop full-range muscle strength (Graves et al. 1989; Jones et al. 1988). Researchers at the University of Florida Medical School showed that persons with low muscle strength in positions of trunk extension were more likely to experience low-back pain. They also discovered that training the low-back muscles through the full movement range markedly increased trunk extension strength and significantly decreased low-back discomfort (Risch et al. 1993).

> **Full-Range Strength Training:** *Performing each repetition through the positions of joint extension and joint flexion as determined by the client's pain-free movement range.*

Performing full-range strength training exercises also may enhance physical performance. Senior golfers who performed full-range strengthening and stretching exercises improved their driving ability (measured by club head speed) by 6% after eight weeks of training, compared to no improvement in those who did not exercise (Westcott et al. 1996).

The term *full-range* implies the performance of an exercise from the position of full muscle stretch to the position of full muscle contraction assuming the client is able to do so. It should be noted that when the targeted muscle group (e.g., quadriceps) is fully contracted, the opposing muscle group (e.g., hamstrings) is fully stretched. Therefore, full-range training simultaneously strengthens as well as stretches the muscle pairs that control joint actions. Such training encourages a good balance of strength across joints and also helps to increase functional movement range in those older adults who have been sedentary.

Although ranges of movement vary among individuals, it is advantageous to perform full-range resistance exercises whenever possible. Exceptions are the free-weight squat, in which full-depth squats are not recommended, as well as any exercise that causes joint discomfort. Training should not cause pain during any phase of movement, and should never exceed normal joint limits. Eliminate exercises that produce immediate or delayed discomfort in the joints, or else abbreviate the range to permit pain-free movement. Do not have older adults exceed a comfortable range of movement—an unnecessary effort at best, since continued training typically results in an extended range of pain-free movement. Chapter 4 provides some helpful suggestions regarding selection and modifications of exercises.

Movement Speed

Movement speed refers to the time required to perform each exercise repetition (i.e., to lift and lower the weight load). Faster speeds generally create more momentum and result in less consistent muscle force production. As momentum increases, so does the risk of injury. Conversely, slower movement speeds create less momentum and more consistent muscle tension throughout the range of movement. Performing repetitions in a slow and controlled manner enhances exercise safety and is recommended for older adult strength training programs. We define a slow and controlled movement speed as a repetition in which two seconds are used during the more difficult concentric muscle action (lifting movement during which the muscle shortens) and four seconds are used during the less demanding eccentric muscle action (lowering movement during which the muscle lengthens).

Athletes often use fast training speeds to improve their performance in competitive sports. There is little justification for older adults to do so, however, unless they too are training for competition. Have your clients perform every repetition under complete control. A simple way to help trainees determine for themselves if they are moving too fast is to administer the *stop test*. Ask them to stop the weightload at a specified point in the movement range. If they can't do so, the movement speed is too fast.

> **Controlled Speed Training:** *Perform each repetition in about 6 seconds, using 2 seconds for the concentric action and 4 during the eccentric phase.*

Exercise Breathing

It is especially important for older adults to breathe properly during exercise. Regardless of the exercise effort, your clients should never hold their breath (referred to as "engaging the Valsalva maneuver") when performing strength training exercises. The Valsalva maneuver produces excessive internal pressure that restricts blood flow back to the heart—contributing to high blood pressure responses and possibly to lightheadedness, dizziness, and even blackouts. By breathing continuously throughout every repetition of an exercise, your clients will avoid these undesirable effects.

> **Proper Breathing:** *Exhale during the more demanding concentric muscle action, and inhale during the less demanding eccentric muscle action.*

Warm-Up and Cooldown

Just as it is important to warm up before and cool down after aerobic activity, senior exercisers should do the same when strength training. The few minutes required for these activities is time well spent.

Warm-Up

Because strength training is a high-effort physical activity that places significant demands on the musculoskeletal system, you should prepare your clients for each workout with a few minutes of warm-up activity. The purpose of the warm-up is to gradually shift the muscular and cardiovascular systems from a resting to a working state. Standard warm-up exercises include walking, cycling, and stepping, followed by a few calisthenic exercises such as knee bends, side bends, and trunk curls. The warm-up period should typically take between 5 and 10 minutes. If there is any concern regarding the readiness of the targeted muscles and joints for a particular exercise, performing a preliminary set with approximately half the training load provides an excellent exercise-specific warm-up. Clients should complete about 10 standard speed repetitions with the lighter load before performing the first set with the assigned weightload.

Cooldown

The cooldown is essentially a warm-up in reverse. It helps the muscular and cardiovascular systems gradually shift from a working to a resting state. The cooldown is particularly important for older adults: blood that accumulates in the lower legs following vigorous exercise can cause undesirable changes in blood pressure and may lead to cardiovascular complications. Five to ten minutes of cooldown activity facilitates a smooth return to resting circulation and blood flow back to the heart. Recommended cooldown exercises include easy walking and cycling, followed by stretching exercises such as those shown on pages 36-37. Although time limitations may tend to crowd the warm-up and cooldown segments, these important transitional activities should be standard procedure in each training session.

Warm-Up and Cooldown: Clients should perform 5 to 10 minutes of light exercise before and after each strength workout to assist the body's transition between resting and exercise states.

Summary of Teaching Strategies and Training Procedures

A successful educational and motivational strategy for older adult exercisers should include

- understandable performance objectives,
- concise instruction with precise demonstration,

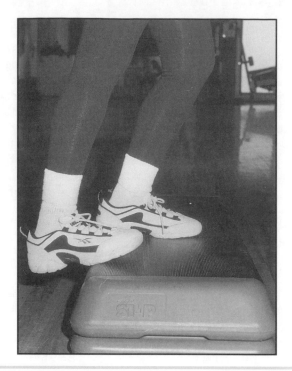

Figure 3.1   Step stretch.

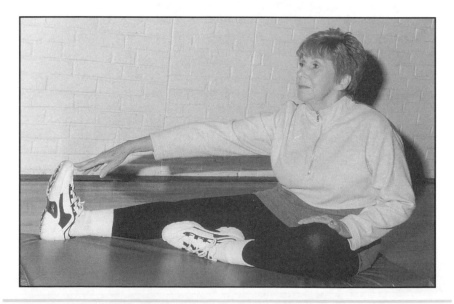

Figure 3.2   Number 4 stretch.

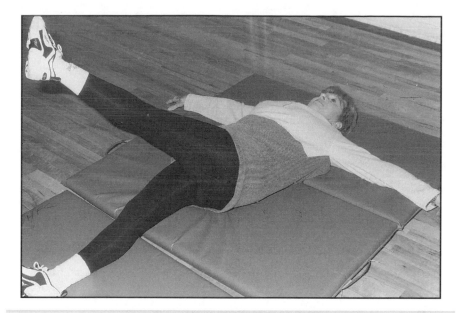

Figure 3.3   Letter T stretch.

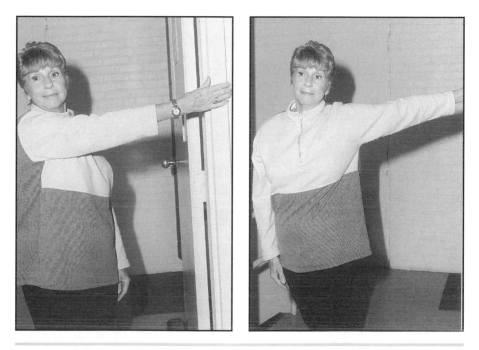

Figure 3.4   Doorway stretch.

- attentive supervision,
- appropriate assistance,
- one task at a time,
- gradual progression,
- positive reinforcement,
- specific feedback,
- careful questioning, and
- pre- and postexercise dialogue.

Pre- and postexercise dialogue should always involve the four key words: hello, goodbye, thank you, and the client's name.

To enhance training effectiveness and reduce injury risk, senior exercisers should perform full-range movements (without experiencing discomfort) at relatively slow movement speeds (six seconds per repetition). Clients should breathe continuously throughout each exercise repetition, exhaling during the concentric muscle action and inhaling during the eccentric muscle action. Older adults should begin each strength training session with a few minutes of warm-up activity, and should conclude their workout with at least five minutes of cooldown exercise.

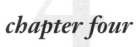

chapter four

Free-Weight and Machine Exercises

Once your clients understand the general procedures for safe and productive strength training, they are ready to learn specific muscle-building exercises. Seniors who train at home typically use free weights, whereas those who train at a fitness facility generally use machines or a combination of machines and free weights.

Free-weight training is inexpensive, requires little space, and offers a wide variety of exercise movements. It is generally considered more technical, however, and therefore requires more competent instruction and careful supervision than does machine-based training to ensure that exercises are performed safely and correctly.

Machine training offers structural support for the body and provides relatively fixed movement patterns, making improper positions less likely. Many machines also have variable resistance features that automatically change resistance according to muscle force capacity in different regions of the movement range. That is, they present proportionately less resistance in weaker muscle positions and proportionately more resistance in stronger muscle positions.

There are alternatives to standard free-weight and machine training, such as training with elastic bands or bodyweight resistance. Selected exercises for seniors using elastic bands and bodyweight resistance are illustrated and described in chapter 7.

Regardless of the equipment used, senior exercisers should observe the guidelines presented on page 41 to maximize their training effectiveness and minimize their risk of injury. For your convenience, we have presented these guidelines as a handout that you may copy and give to your clients. To achieve a full 8.5" × 11" form, copy it at 145%.

This chapter provides photo illustrations (beginning and ending positions) of recommended machine and free-weight exercises for senior strength trainers. We also present verbal instructions you may give your clients, potential problems you may encounter, and suggestions for safely overcoming these obstacles.

Strength Exercises for Machine and Free-Weight Training

The following exercises are organized into three major sections: those that work the lower body muscles, those that address the midsection muscles, and those that target muscles of the upper body. The exercises are further categorized by the specific muscles involved, such as the quadriceps, rectus abdominis, pectoralis major, etc. The anatomical drawings in figures 4.1a and b present names and locations of the major muscles for convenient cross-referencing with the exercise descriptions.

Due to predisposing factors such as previous illness, injury, or musculo-skeletal weakness, many older adults require modifications in their strength training programs. Specific conditions (obesity, diabetes, cardiovascular disease, etc.) and training recommendations are discussed in chapter 8. The exercise descriptions in this section include common training problems for healthy seniors, along with suggested modifications that should enable them to successfully perform the movements. *Important:* Exercises in which the trainee could be pinned underneath a barbell, such as barbell bench presses and squats, *must* be performed with a spotter as indicated in the training guidelines. Refer clients with significant or persistent pain to a qualified medical professional for proper evaluation and treatment before they continue in the training program. The following recommendations for rating and remediating pain were developed by Dr. Ben Kibler (Penn State Sports Medicine Newsletter 1997) and may prove helpful with clients who experience training discomfort:

- **Level 1:** Pain that hurts after exercise, but subsides by the next day.

  Treatment: Stretch after exercise; apply ice; take ibuprofen.

- **Level 2:** Pain that develops during exercise but does not interfere with one's ability to continue.

  Treatment: Same as Level 1 treatment; also reduce the intensity of exercise to prevent further injury.

- **Level 3:** Pain that occurs throughout an exercise period and interferes with one's ability to participate.

  Treatment: Seek a medical evaluation and treatment immediately.

Guidelines for Safe and Effective Exercise

- Use full-range exercise movements.

- Use moderate to slow movement speeds.

- Breathe throughout every repetition, exhaling when lifting the weight and inhaling when lowering the weight.

- Perform a few minutes of warm-up activity before and a few minutes of cooldown activity after each strength workout.

- Set the seat position, pin the weightstack, and secure the seat belt (when provided) before doing machine exercises.

- Load the bar evenly, secure the collars, and check equipment stability (bench, squat rack, etc.) before doing free-weight exercises.

- Train with a spotter when doing barbell bench presses or barbell squats.

- Record exercise weightloads, repetitions, sets, and other relevant training information on the workout cards.

- Train within your present ability level, always ending the exercise set before proper performance technique is compromised.

- Reduce the resistance in any exercise that feels too stressful.

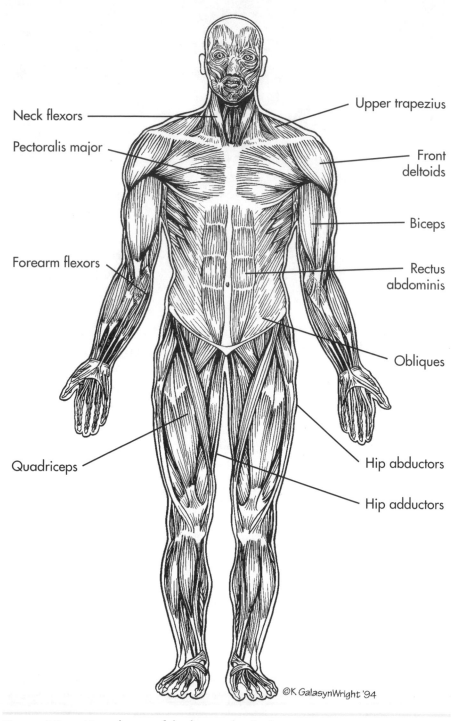

Neck flexors

Upper trapezius

Pectoralis major

Front deltoids

Biceps

Forearm flexors

Rectus abdominis

Obliques

Quadriceps

Hip abductors

Hip adductors

©K GalasynWright '94

Figure 4.1a   Musculature of the human body, front.
© K. Galasyn-Wright, Champaign, IL, 1994

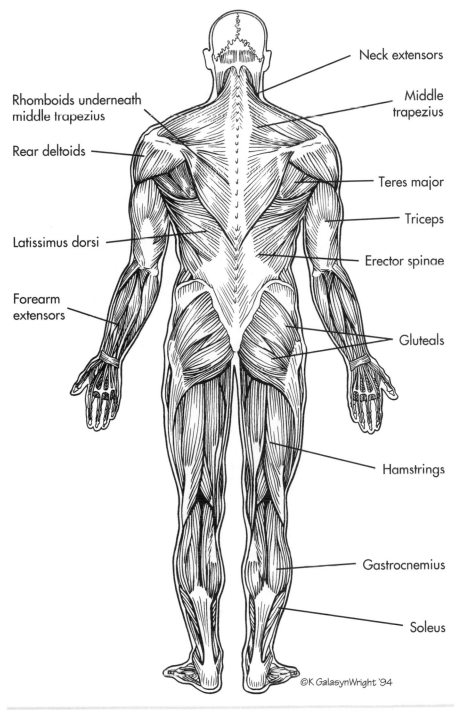

Neck extensors

Rhomboids underneath middle trapezius

Middle trapezius

Rear deltoids

Teres major

Triceps

Latissimus dorsi

Erector spinae

Forearm extensors

Gluteals

Hamstrings

Gastrocnemius

Soleus

©K GalasynWright '94

Figure 4.1b   Musculature of the human body, back.
© K. Galasyn-Wright, Champaign, IL, 1994

- **Level 4:** Pain that persists even after training sessions and severely restricts participation in physical activity.

Treatment: Seek a medical evaluation and treatment immediately.

Lower Body Exercises

Below you will find 10 exercises for the lower body. These include exercises for strengthening the legs, hips, and calves.

MACHINE LEG EXTENSION

Quadriceps

DIRECTIONS FOR YOUR CLIENT

Beginning Position

1. Adjust seat so knees are in line with machine's axis of rotation (where machine pivots).
2. Sit with back firmly against seat pad.
3. Position ankles behind roller pad, knees flexed about 90 degrees.
4. Grip handles.

Upward Movement Phase

1. Push roller pad slowly upward until knees are extended.
2. Exhale throughout upward movement.

Downward Movement Phase

1. Slowly return roller pad to starting position.
2. Inhale throughout lowering movement.

POSSIBLE PROBLEMS AND RECOMMENDED MODIFICATIONS

- *Knee pain, particularly in positions of knee flexion*
  Double pin the weightstack by placing weightstack in desired range of movement with the first pin and locking into place with the second pin, or use built-in range limiter to restrict action to the pain-free range of movement.

- *Inability to reach full knee extension*
  Use lighter weightload to permit greater movement range.

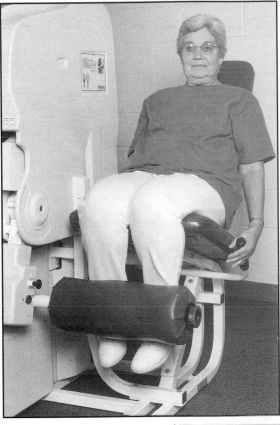

Beginning position.

Upward movement phase.

MACHINE LEG CURL

Hamstrings

DIRECTIONS FOR YOUR CLIENT

Beginning Position

1. Adjust seat so knee joint is in line with machine's axis of rotation.
2. Sit with back firmly against seat pad.
3. Position lower legs between roller pads, knees extended.
4. Grip handles.

Backward Movement Phase

1. Pull roller pads slowly backward until knees are fully flexed.
2. Exhale throughout pulling movement.

Forward Movement Phase

1. Allow roller pads to return slowly to starting position.
2. Inhale throughout return movement.

POSSIBLE PROBLEMS AND RECOMMENDED MODIFICATIONS

- *Inability to reach full knee flexion*
  Use lighter weightload to permit greater movement range.

- *Discomfort in low back in positions of knee flexion*
  Contract abdominal muscles to maintain flat back contact with seatback.

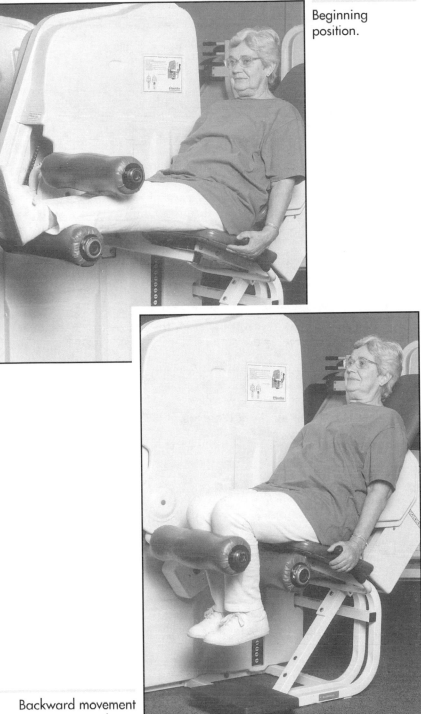

Beginning
position.

Backward movement
phase.

FREE-WEIGHT DUMBBELL SQUAT

Quadriceps, Hamstrings, Gluteals

DIRECTIONS FOR YOUR CLIENT

Beginning Position

1. Grasp dumbbells and stand erect with feet about hip-width apart and parallel to each other.
2. Position dumbbells with palms facing outer thighs.
3. Keep head up, eyes fixed straight ahead, shoulders back, back straight, and weight on entire foot throughout the upward and downward movement phases of this exercise.

Downward Movement Phase

1. Slowly squat down until thighs are parallel to floor.
2. Inhale throughout downward movement.
3. If balance is a problem, try positioning your upper back and buttocks against a wall for support (i.e., slide up and down a wall).

Upward Movement Phase

1. Begin upward movement by slowly straightening the knees and hips.
2. Exhale throughout upward movement.

POSSIBLE PROBLEMS AND RECOMMENDED MODIFICATIONS

- *Knee pain in lower squat positions*
  Abbreviate descent to permit pain-free squat action.

- *Excess tension on knees, feet, and Achilles tendon as indicated by heels lifting off floor*
  With chest out, move hips backward as well as downward on descent to keep knees directly above feet and heels flat on floor. Also, try widening the stance.

- *Discomfort in shoulders, arms, or hands*
  Hold dumbbells on shoulders rather than beside hips.

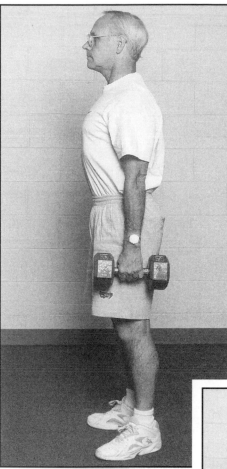

Beginning position.

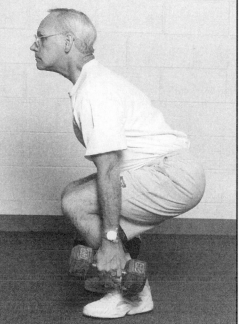

Downward movement phase.

FREE-WEIGHT BARBELL SQUAT

Note: This exercise requires a spotter for safe performance.

Quadriceps, Hamstrings, Gluteals

DIRECTIONS FOR YOUR CLIENT

Beginning Position

1. Position feet shoulder-width apart or wider and grip the bar overhand while it's on a rack.
2. Position bar on shoulders at base of neck, and stand erect.
3. Keep head up, eyes fixed straight ahead, shoulders back, back straight, and weight on entire foot throughout the upward and downward movement phases of this exercise.

Downward Movement Phase

1. Slowly squat down until thighs are parallel to floor.
2. Inhale throughout downward movement.

Upward Movement Phase

1. Begin upward movement by slowly straightening knees and hips.
2. Exhale throughout upward movement.
3. Carefully return the bar to rack after completing the set.

POSSIBLE PROBLEMS AND RECOMMENDED MODIFICATIONS

- *Knee pain in lower squat positions*
  Abbreviate descent to permit pain-free squat action.

- *Stress on knees, feet, and Achilles tendons as indicated by heels lifting off floor*
  With chest out, move hips backward as well as downward on descent to keep knees directly above feet and heels flat on floor. Also, try widening the stance.

- *Discomfort in shoulders, neck, or back*
  Reposition barbell so that it rests farther back on trapezius muscle, use wider hand spacing, or switch to dumbbell squats.

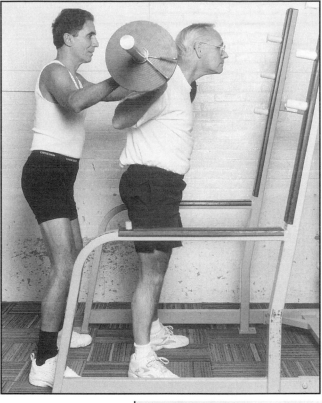

Beginning position.

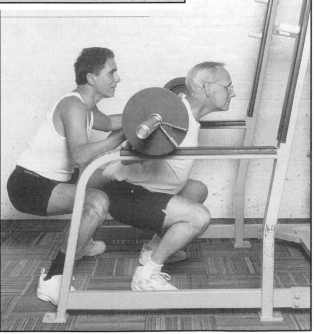

Downward movement
phase.

MACHINE LEG PRESS

Quadriceps, Hamstrings, Gluteals

DIRECTIONS FOR YOUR CLIENT

Beginning Position

1. Adjust seat so knees are flexed to 90 degrees or less.
2. Sit with back firmly against seat pad.
3. Place feet flat on foot pad, in line with knees and hips.
4. Grip handles with hands.

Forward Movement Phase

1. Slowly push foot pad forward until knees are almost extended, but not locked.
2. Keep feet, knees, and hips aligned.
3. Exhale throughout pushing phase.

Backward Movement Phase

1. Allow foot pad to slowly return to starting position.
2. Inhale throughout return movement.

POSSIBLE PROBLEMS AND RECOMMENDED MODIFICATIONS

- *Knee pain in various positions of knee extension*
  Keep knees directly behind feet and same width as hips. Do not flex knees beyond 90 degrees in rear position, and stop short of lockout in forward position.

- *Hip or groin pain in positions of hip flexion*
  Limit hip flexion to pain-free range of movement; usually consistent with 90 degrees of knee flexion.

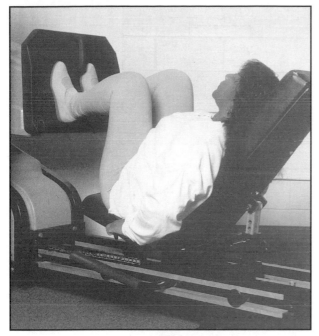

Beginning position.

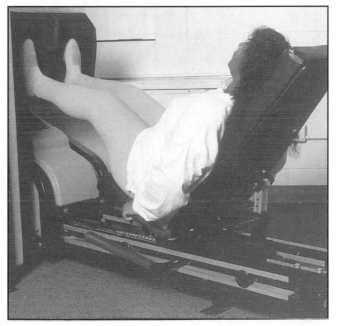

Forward movement phase.

MACHINE HIP ADDUCTION

Hip Adductors

DIRECTIONS FOR YOUR CLIENT

Beginning Position

1. Sit with back firmly against seat pad.
2. Position knees outside of movement pads and ankles on supports.
3. Adjust movement lever to starting position with legs comfortably apart.
4. Grip handles with hands.

Inward Movement Phase

1. Slowly pull movement pads together.
2. Exhale throughout pulling movement.

Outward Movement Phase

1. Allow pads to slowly return to starting position with legs apart.
2. Inhale throughout return movement.

POSSIBLE PROBLEMS AND RECOMMENDED MODIFICATIONS

- *Pain or pressure in knee area*
  Reposition seat or add a back pad so that the movement pads contact the thighs rather than the knees.

- *Pain in hip area*
  Reduce range of leg separation to permit pain-free movements.

- *Pain in low back*
  Contract abdominal muscles to maintain flat back contact with seatback.

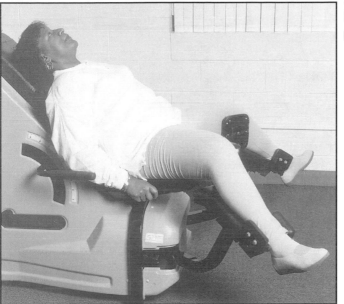

Beginning
position.

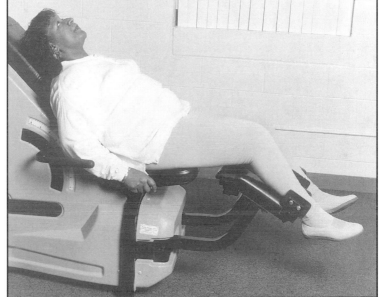

Inward
movement
phase.

MACHINE HIP ABDUCTION

Hip Abductors

DIRECTIONS FOR YOUR CLIENT

Beginning Position

1. Sit with back firmly against seat pad.
2. Position knees inside of movement pads and ankles on supports, with legs together.
3. Grip handles with hands.

Outward Movement Phase

1. Slowly push movement pads apart as far as comfortable.
2. Exhale throughout pushing movement.

Inward Movement Phase

1. Allow movement pads to slowly return to starting position with legs together.
2. Inhale throughout return movement.

POSSIBLE PROBLEMS AND RECOMMENDED MODIFICATIONS

- *Pain or pressure in knee area*
  Reposition seat or add a back pad so that the movement pads contact the thighs rather than the knees.

- *Pain in groin area*
  Reduce range of leg separation to permit pain-free movements.

- *Pain in low back*
  Contract abdominal muscles to maintain flat back contact with seatback.

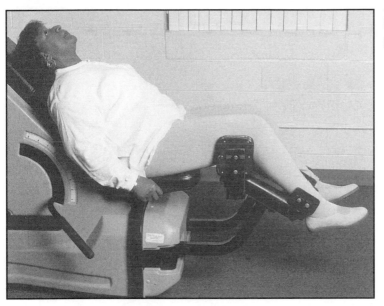

Beginning
position.

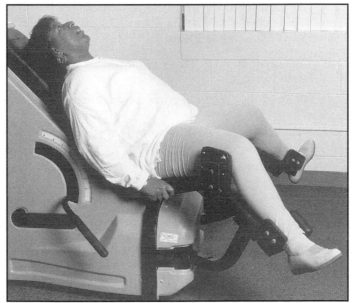

Outward
movement
phase.

FREE-WEIGHT DUMBBELL HEEL RAISE

Gastrocnemius, Soleus

DIRECTIONS FOR YOUR CLIENT

Beginning Position

1. Grasp dumbbells with an overhand grip and stand erect.
2. Position dumbbells with palms facing outer thighs.
3. Place balls of feet on a *stable*, elevated surface (approximately four inches high), feet hip-width apart and parallel to each other.
4. Keep head up, eyes fixed straight ahead, shoulders back, back straight, and weight on balls of the feet throughout the upward and downward movement phases of this exercise.

Upward Movement Phase

1. Rise up slowly on the toes while keeping torso erect and knees straight.
2. Exhale throughout upward movement.

Downward Movement Phase

1. Lower the heels as far as comfortable while keeping torso erect and knees straight.
2. Inhale throughout lowering movement.

POSSIBLE PROBLEMS AND RECOMMENDED MODIFICATIONS

- *Low back discomfort*
  Maintain erect posture throughout exercise.

- *Discomfort in shoulders, arms, or hands*
  Hold dumbbells on shoulders rather than beside hips.

- *Strain in calf muscles or Achilles tendons*
  Decrease distance heels are lowered below board.

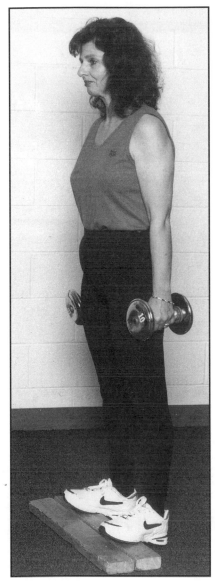

Beginning position.

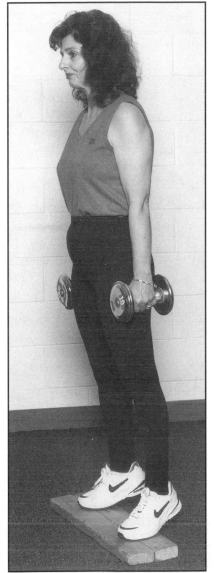

Upward movement phase.

FREE-WEIGHT BARBELL HEEL RAISE

Gastrocnemius, Soleus

DIRECTIONS FOR YOUR CLIENT

Beginning Position

1. Position feet shoulder-width apart and grip the bar overhand while it's on a rack.
2. Hold bar against thighs with arms straight, head up, and eyes looking ahead.
3. Stand erect.
4. Place balls of feet on a *stable*, elevated surface (approximately four inches high), feet hip-width apart and parallel to each other.
5. Keep head up, eyes fixed straight ahead, shoulders back, back straight, and weight on balls of feet throughout the upward and downward movement phases of this exercise.

Upward Movement Phase

1. Slowly rise on toes while keeping torso erect and knees straight.
2. Exhale throughout upward movement.

Downward Movement Phase

1. Lower the heels as far as comfortable while keeping torso erect and knees straight.
2. Inhale throughout lowering movement.
3. Carefully return bar to rack.

POSSIBLE PROBLEMS AND RECOMMENDED MODIFICATIONS

- *Low back discomfort*
  Maintain erect posture throughout exercise.

- *Discomfort in shoulders, neck, or back*
  Place barbell so that it rests farther back on trapezius muscle similar to barbell squat position.

- *Strain in feet or Achilles tendons*
  Decrease distance heels are lowered below board.

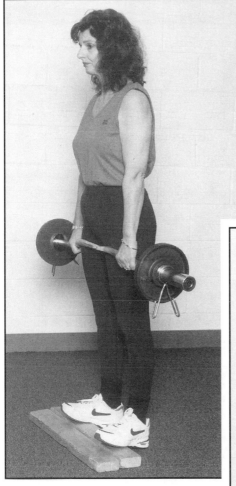

Beginning position.

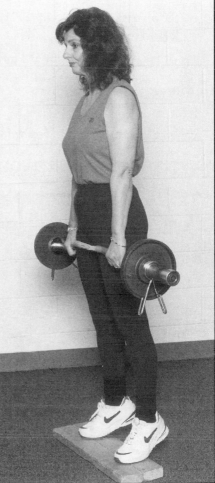

Upward movement phase.

MACHINE HEEL RAISE

Gastrocnemius, Soleus

DIRECTIONS FOR YOUR CLIENT

Beginning Position

1. Position and secure the resistance belt around waist.
2. Stand with balls of feet on rear edge of step.
3. Place hands on support bar.
4. Allow heels to drop below step as far as comfortable.

Upward Movement Phase

1. Slowly rise on toes to lift heels upward as high as possible.
2. Keep knees straight.
3. Exhale throughout upward movement.

Downward Movement Phase

1. Return slowly to starting position, heels below step.
2. Inhale throughout downward movement.

POSSIBLE PROBLEMS AND RECOMMENDED MODIFICATIONS

- *Low back discomfort*
  Reposition resistance belt to a more comfortable position, and maintain erect posture throughout exercise.

- *Strain in feet or Achilles tendons*
  Decrease distance heels are lowered below step.

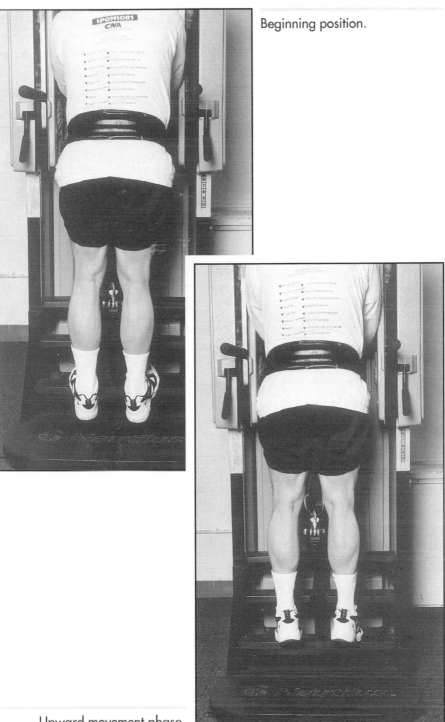

Beginning position.

Upward movement phase.

Midsection Exercises

Below you will find five exercises that address the midsection of the body. These include exercises for strengthening the low-back, abdominal, and oblique muscles.

MACHINE BACK EXTENSION

Erector Spinae

DIRECTIONS FOR YOUR CLIENT

Beginning Position

1. Sit all the way back on seat and adjust foot pad so knees are slightly higher than hips.
2. Secure seat belt across thighs and hips.
3. Cross arms on chest.
4. Place upper back firmly against pad with trunk flexed forward.

Backward Movement Phase

1. Push upper back against pad until trunk is fully extended.
2. Keep head in line with torso.
3. Exhale throughout extension movement.

Forward Movement Phase

1. Slowly return pad to starting position.
2. Inhale throughout return movement.

POSSIBLE PROBLEMS AND RECOMMENDED MODIFICATIONS

- *Discomfort in low back area*
  Abbreviate trunk extension to pain-free range of movement.

- *Strain in neck area*
  Maintain neutral head position throughout exercise.

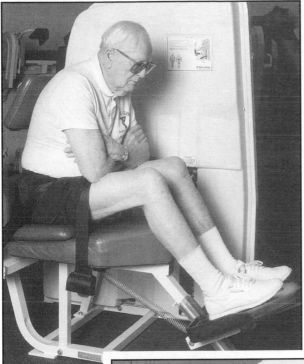

Beginning position.

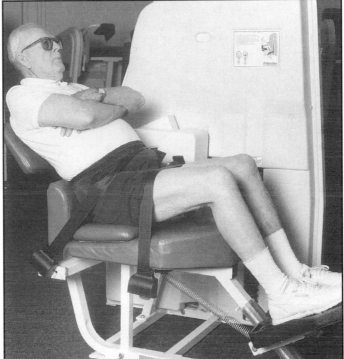

Backward
movement phase.

FREE-WEIGHT BACK EXTENSION

Erector Spinae

DIRECTIONS FOR YOUR CLIENT

Beginning Position

1. Lie face down on mat or carpeted floor.
2. Place hands loosely behind head.
3. A weight plate may be held behind the head for added resistance.

Upward Movement Phase

1. Slowly raise chest about 30 degrees off floor until low-back muscles are fully contracted.
2. Keep hips on floor at all times.
3. Exhale throughout upward movement.

Downward Movement Phase

1. Slowly lower chest to floor.
2. Inhale throughout lowering movement.

POSSIBLE PROBLEMS AND RECOMMENDED MODIFICATIONS

- *Inability to lift chest off floor*
  Secure feet to provide an anchor for trunk extension movement. Place hands by shoulders and use arms to assist the low-back muscles as in a modified push-up.

- *Discomfort in low back area*
  Limit lifting action to the pain-free range of movement. Place hands by shoulders and use arms to assist the low-back muscles, as in a modified push-up.

- *Strain in neck area*
  Maintain neutral head position throughout exercise.

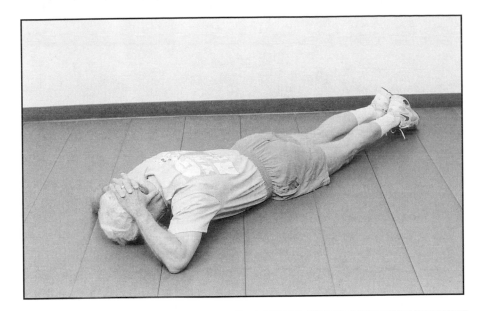

Beginning position.

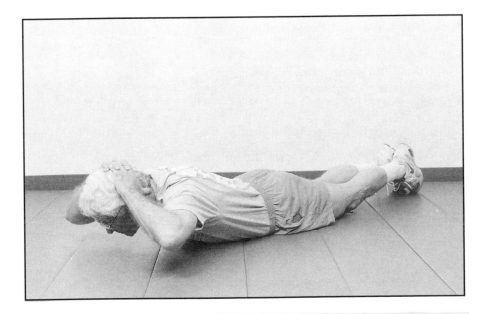

Upward movement phase.

MACHINE ABDOMINAL CURL

Rectus Abdominis

DIRECTIONS FOR YOUR CLIENT

Beginning Position

1. Adjust seat so navel is aligned with machine's axis of rotation.
2. Secure seat belt.
3. Sit with upper back firmly against pad.
4. Place elbows on arm pads and hands on handles.

Forward Movement Phase

1. Slowly pull pad forward until trunk is fully flexed by contracting abdominal muscles (tightening abdominal muscles as tight as you can get them).
2. Keep upper back firmly against pad.
3. Exhale throughout forward movement.

Backward Movement Phase

1. Slowly return pad to starting position.
2. Inhale throughout return movement.

POSSIBLE PROBLEMS AND RECOMMENDED MODIFICATIONS

- *Discomfort in low back area*
  Abbreviate trunk flexion to pain-free range of movement.

- *Strain in neck area*
  Maintain neutral head position throughout exercise.

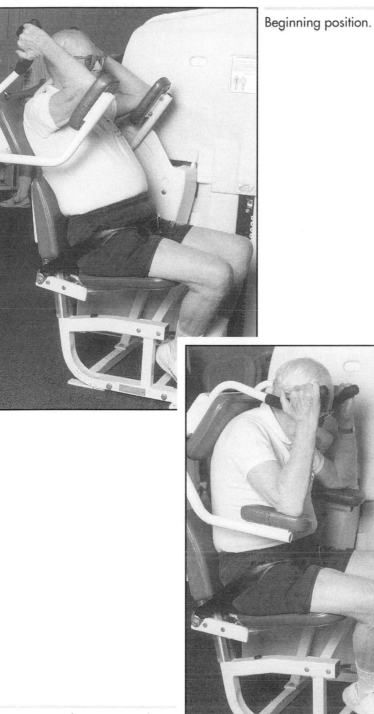

Beginning position.

Forward movement phase.

FREE-WEIGHT TRUNK CURL

Rectus Abdominis

DIRECTIONS FOR YOUR CLIENT

Beginning Position

1. Lie on back on mat or carpeted floor.
2. Flex knees to 110 degrees, feet flat on the floor.
3. Place hands loosely behind head to maintain neutral neck position.
4. A weight plate may be held behind the head for added resistance.

Upward Movement Phase

1. Slowly raise shoulders about 30 degrees off floor until abdominal muscles are fully contracted.
2. Exhale throughout upward movement.

Downward Movement Phase

1. Slowly lower shoulders to floor.
2. Inhale throughout lowering movement.

POSSIBLE PROBLEMS AND RECOMMENDED MODIFICATIONS

- *Discomfort in low back area*
  Bring feet closer to hips to increase hip flexion and decrease arch in low-back area.

- *Strain in neck area*
  Maintain neutral head position throughout exercise.

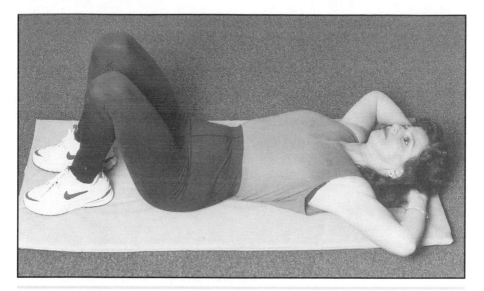

Beginning position.

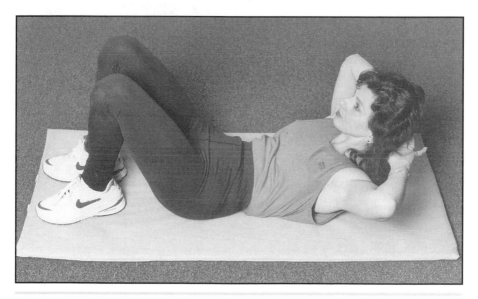

Upward movement phase.

MACHINE ROTARY TORSO

Rectus Abdominis, External Obliques, Internal Obliques

DIRECTIONS FOR YOUR CLIENT

Beginning Position

1. Sit all the way back on seat with torso erect, facing forward.
2. Wrap legs around seat extension.
3. Position upper arms against arm pads.

Left Movement Phase

1. Turn torso slowly to left, about 45 degrees.
2. Exhale throughout rotation.

Return Movement Phase

1. Slowly return torso to starting position (facing forward).
2. Inhale throughout return movement.
3. Change seat position and repeat exercise to right.

POSSIBLE PROBLEMS AND RECOMMENDED MODIFICATIONS

- *Discomfort in shoulders, midsection, or hips*
  Reduce torso turning distance to pain-free range of movement.

- *Pressure in arms*
  Place equal emphasis on both arms by repositioning so that one arm pulls and one arm pushes the arm pads.

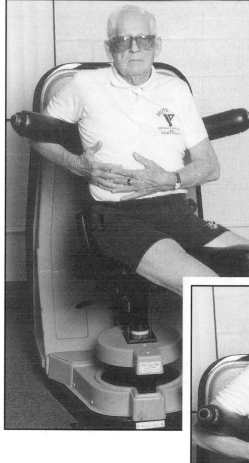

Beginning position.

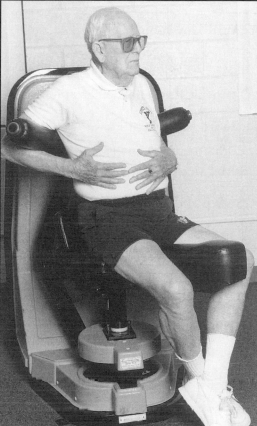

Left movement phase.

Upper Body Exercises

Below you will find 25 exercises that address the upper body. These include exercises for strengthening the pectorals, upper back, shoulders, and arms.

MACHINE CHEST CROSSOVER

Pectoralis Major, Anterior Deltoid

DIRECTIONS FOR YOUR CLIENT

Beginning Position

1. Adjust seat so shoulders are in line with machine's axes of rotation and upper arms are parallel to floor.
2. Sit with head, shoulders, and back firmly against seat pad.
3. Position forearms against arm pads and hands on handles.

Forward Movement Phase

1. Pull arm pads slowly together, using arms more than hands.
2. Keep wrists straight.
3. Exhale throughout pulling movement.

Backward Movement Phase

1. Slowly return arm pads to starting position.
2. Inhale throughout return movement.

POSSIBLE PROBLEMS AND RECOMMENDED MODIFICATIONS

- *Pain in shoulders or strain in chest area*
  Reduce backwards movement range so that hands are always in front of shoulders.

- *Discomfort in elbow area*
  Reposition seat or add a back pad so that the movement pads make greater contact with arms.

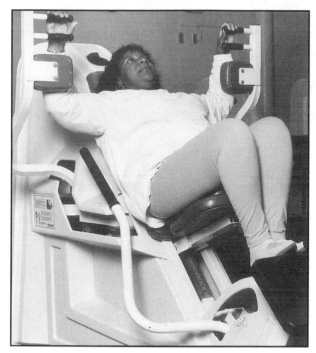

Beginning position.

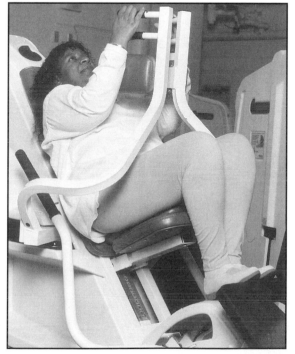

Forward movement phase.

FREE-WEIGHT DUMBBELL CHEST FLY

Pectoralis Major, Anterior Deltoid

DIRECTIONS FOR YOUR CLIENT

Beginning Position

1. Lie on back on bench with legs straddling bench and knees flexed at 90 degrees, feet flat on the floor.
2. Keep head, shoulders, and buttocks in contact with the bench and feet in contact with the floor throughout exercise.
3. Grasp dumbbells so palms face each other.
4. Push dumbbells in unison to a position over chest with elbows slightly flexed.

Downward Movement Phase

1. Slowly lower dumbbells in unison, keeping elbows slightly flexed and perpendicular to torso.
2. Continue lowering dumbbells until upper arms are parallel to floor.
3. Inhale throughout lowering movement.

Upward Movement Phase

1. Lift dumbbells upward in unison to the starting position (elbows slightly flexed).
2. Exhale throughout upward movement.

POSSIBLE PROBLEMS AND RECOMMENDED MODIFICATIONS

- *Pain in shoulders or strain in chest area*
  Reduce downward movement range so that hands are always above shoulder level.

- *Discomfort in elbow area*
  Keep elbows comfortably flexed throughout each repetition.

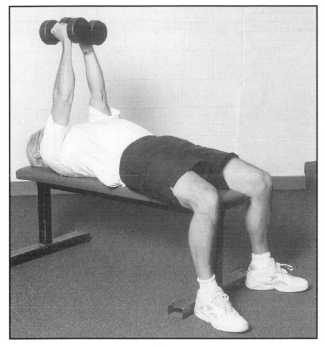

Beginning position.

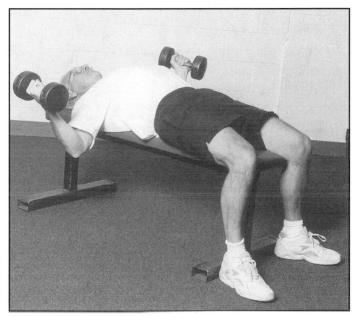

Downward
movement
phase.

MACHINE CHEST PRESS

Pectoralis Major, Anterior Deltoid, Triceps

DIRECTIONS FOR YOUR CLIENT

Beginning Position

1. Adjust seat so handles are right below shoulder level.
2. Sit with head, shoulders, and back against seat pad.
3. Place feet on foot pad and press forward to bring handles into starting position by chest.
4. Grasp handles with fingers and thumbs.
5. Release foot pad slowly.

Forward Movement Phase

1. Push handles forward slowly until arms are fully extended.
2. Keep wrists straight.
3. Exhale throughout pushing movement.

Backward Movement Phase

1. Slowly return handles to the starting position.
2. Inhale throughout the return phase.
3. After completing the final repetition, place feet on foot pad, press forward to hold weightstack, release hand grips, and lower weightstack slowly.

POSSIBLE PROBLEMS AND RECOMMENDED MODIFICATIONS

- *Pain in shoulders*
  Reduce backwards movement range so that hands are always in front of chest.

- *Discomfort in low back area*
  Contract abdominals to maintain flat back contact with seatback.

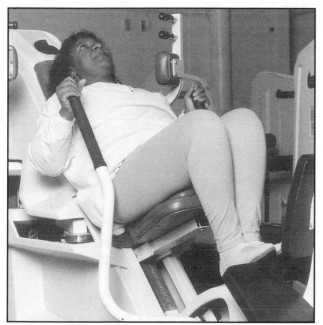

Beginning position.

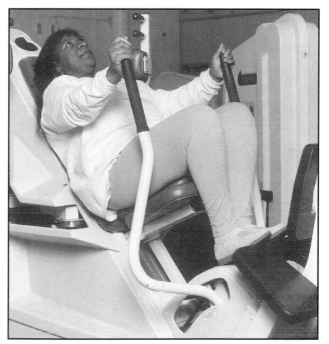

Forward movement
phase.

FREE-WEIGHT DUMBBELL BENCH PRESS

Pectoralis Major, Anterior Deltoid, Triceps

DIRECTIONS FOR YOUR CLIENT

Beginning Position

1. Lie on back with legs straddling bench, knees flexed at 90 degrees, feet flat on floor.
2. Keep head, shoulders, and buttocks in contact with the bench and feet in contact with the floor throughout the exercise.
3. Grasp dumbbells so palms face away, and push upwards until arms are fully extended above chest.

Downward Movement Phase

1. Slowly lower dumbbells in unison to the outsides of chest.
2. Inhale throughout lowering movement.

Upward Movement Phase

1. Press dumbbells upward in unison until arms are fully extended.
2. Exhale throughout upward movement.

POSSIBLE PROBLEMS AND RECOMMENDED MODIFICATIONS

- *Pain in shoulders*
  Reduce downward movement range and keep dumbbells above shoulders throughout each repetition.

- *Discomfort in low back area*
  Place feet on stool to increase hip flexion and decrease arch in low back.

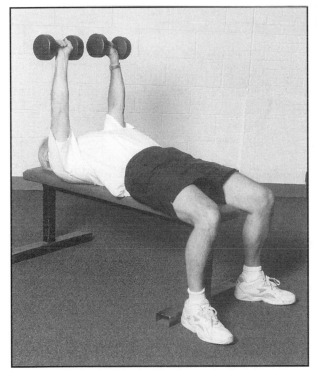

Beginning position.

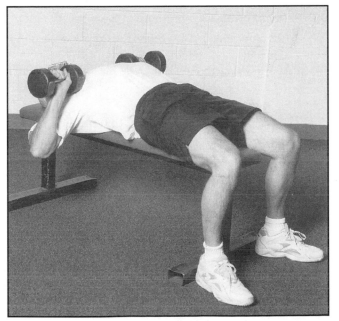

Downward
movement phase.

FREE-WEIGHT BARBELL BENCH PRESS

NOTE: This exercise requires a spotter for safe performance.

Pectoralis Major, Anterior Deltoid, Triceps

DIRECTIONS FOR YOUR CLIENT

Beginning Position

1. With barbell resting on supports, lie on back with legs straddling bench, knees flexed at 90 degrees, feet flat on floor.
2. Keep head, shoulders, and buttocks in contact with the bench, and feet in contact with the floor throughout the exercise.
3. Grasp barbell on supports so palms face away, and push upward until arms are fully extended above chest.

Downward Movement Phase

1. Slowly and evenly lower bar to nipple area of chest.
2. Inhale throughout the lowering movement.

Upward Movement Phase

1. Press bar upward evenly until arms are fully extended.
2. Exhale throughout pressing movement.
3. After completing final repetition replace barbell onto supports.

POSSIBLE PROBLEMS AND RECOMMENDED MODIFICATIONS

- *Pain in shoulders or elbows*
  Replace barbell bench press with dumbbell bench press.

- *Discomfort in low back area*
  Place feet on stool to increase hip flexion and decrease arch in low back.

- *Pain in wrists*
  Adjust hand spacing on barbell to just slightly wider than shoulder width, and keep wrists in neutral position.

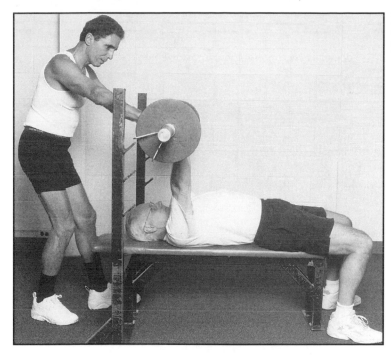

Beginning position.

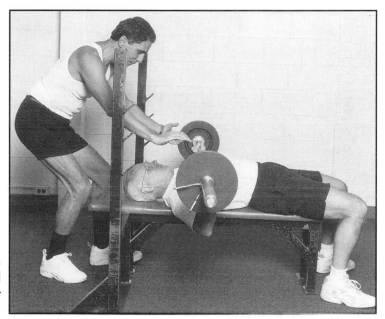

Downward movement phase.

MACHINE WEIGHT-ASSISTED BAR-DIP

Pectoralis Major, Triceps, Anterior Deltoid

DIRECTIONS FOR YOUR CLIENT

Beginning Position

1. Keep in mind that adding weights makes this exercise easier because they counterbalance the bodyweight.
2. Climb steps and grasp dip bars with an overhand grip.
3. Place knees on platform and descend until elbows are flexed about 90 degrees.

Upward Movement Phase

1. Slowly push body upward until arms are fully extended.
2. Keep wrists straight.
3. Keep back straight.
4. Exhale throughout pushing movement.

Downward Movement Phase

1. Return slowly to starting position (until elbows are flexed about 90 degrees).
2. Inhale throughout return movement.

POSSIBLE PROBLEMS AND RECOMMENDED MODIFICATIONS

- *Pain in shoulders*
  Restrict lowering movement to less than 90 degrees of elbow flexion.

- *Discomfort in low back area*
  Maintain erect posture throughout each repetition without arching the back.

- *Pain in wrists*
  Keep wrists in neutral position at all times.

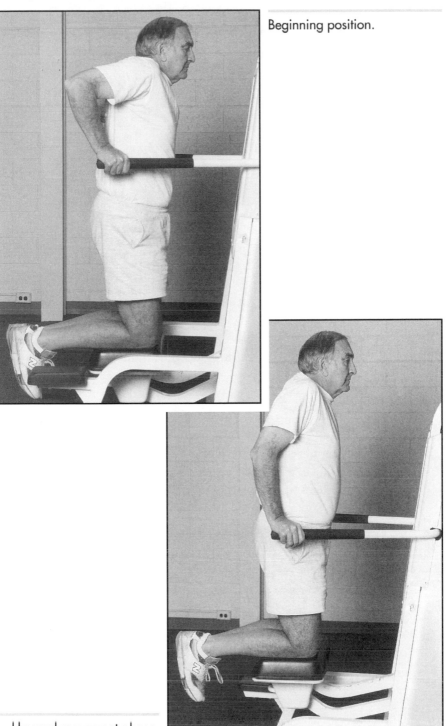

Beginning position.

Upward movement phase.

85

MACHINE SUPER PULLOVER

Latissimus Dorsi

DIRECTIONS FOR YOUR CLIENT

Beginning Position

1. Adjust seat so shoulders are in line with machine's axis of rotation.
2. Sit with back firmly against seat pad, seat belt secured.
3. Place feet on foot lever and press forward to bring arm pads into starting position by face.
4. Position arms against arm pads and hands on bar.
5. Release foot pad.

Downward Movement Phase

1. Slowly pull arm pads downward, using arms more than hands, until bar touches body.
2. Keep wrists straight.
3. Allow back to round slightly during downward movement.
4. Exhale throughout downward movement.

Upward Movement Phase

1. Slowly return arm pads to starting position.
2. Inhale throughout return movement.
3. After completing the final repetition, place feet on foot lever, press forward to hold weightstack, remove arms, and lower weightstack slowly.

POSSIBLE PROBLEMS AND RECOMMENDED MODIFICATIONS

- *Pain in shoulders*
  Reduce backward movement to the pain-free range of exercise action.

- *Discomfort in low back area*
  Contract abdominal muscles during downward movement to flatten back against seatback when movement pads are below shoulder level.

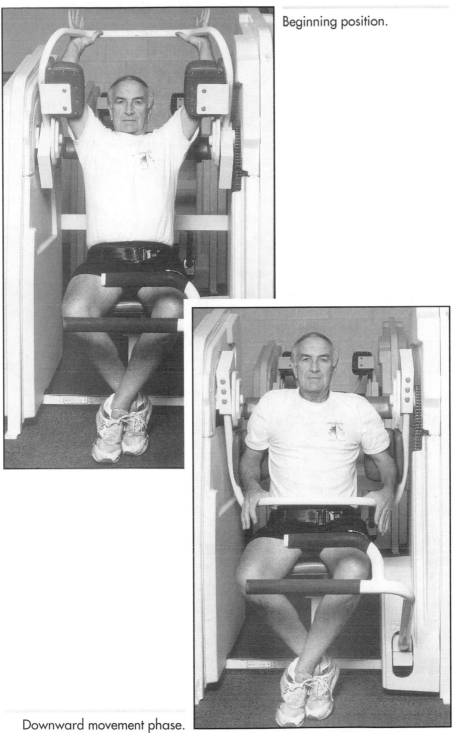

Beginning position.

Downward movement phase.

FREE-WEIGHT DUMBBELL ONE-ARM ROW

Latissimus Dorsi, Biceps

DIRECTIONS FOR YOUR CLIENT

Beginning Position

1. Grasp dumbbell with right hand and support body weight by placing left arm and knee on the bench, keeping the right leg straight and right foot flat on floor.
2. Position dumbbell so that palm faces bench, with arm straight.
3. Keep back flat throughout exercise.

Upward Movement Phase

1. Slowly pull dumbbell to chest.
2. Exhale throughout pulling movement.

Downward Movement Phase

1. Slowly lower dumbbell to starting position.
2. Inhale throughout lowering movement.
3. Repeat exercise from beginning position with left arm.

POSSIBLE PROBLEMS AND RECOMMENDED MODIFICATIONS

- *Pain in shoulder area*
  Keep upper arm close to side throughout exercise, and do not allow shoulder to be pulled downward.

- *Discomfort in low back area*
  Place knee directly under hip and hand directly under shoulder to provide solid base of back support. Keep back and shoulders level throughout each repetition.

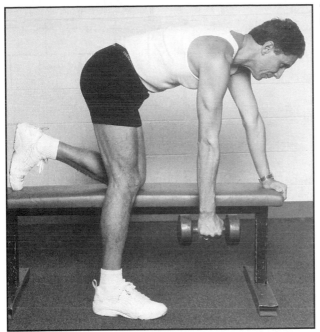

Beginning position.

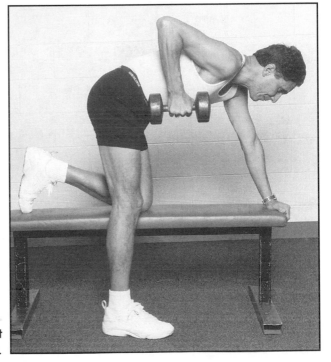

Upward movement
phase.

MACHINE COMPOUND ROW

Latissimus Dorsi, Biceps

DIRECTIONS FOR YOUR CLIENT

Beginning Position

1. Adjust seat so handles are at shoulder level.
2. Sit with chest against chest pad and torso erect.
3. Place feet flat on floor.
4. Grasp each handle, arms fully extended.

Backward Movement Phase

1. Slowly pull handles back toward chest.
2. Keep wrists straight.
3. Exhale throughout pulling movement.

Forward Movement Phase

1. Slowly return handles until arms are fully extended.
2. Inhale throughout return movement.

POSSIBLE PROBLEMS AND RECOMMENDED MODIFICATIONS

- *Discomfort in shoulder area*
  Abbreviate exercise action to pain-free movement range, and do not allow shoulders to be pulled forward.

- *Discomfort in low back area*
  Keep chest in contact with support pad throughout each repetition, particularly at the end of the pulling movements.

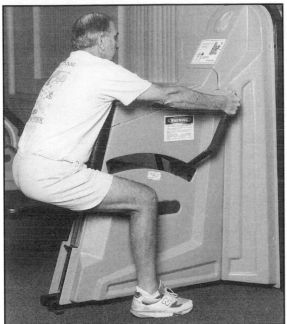

Beginning position.

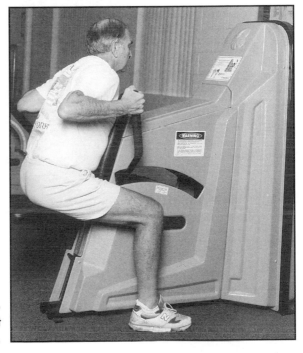

Backward movement
phase.

MACHINE LAT PULLDOWN

Latissimus Dorsi, Biceps

DIRECTIONS FOR YOUR CLIENT

Beginning Position

1. Place knees under restraining pads, keeping torso upright.
2. Grip the bar with hands shoulder-width apart, arms straight, and palms toward face.

Downward Movement Phase

1. Slowly pull bar downward below chin.
2. Exhale throughout pulling movement.

Upward Movement Phase

1. Be prepared for an unexpected upward pull from the bar during the upward movement phase!
2. Slowly return bar to starting position (until arms are fully extended).
3. Inhale throughout the upward movement.

POSSIBLE PROBLEMS AND RECOMMENDED MODIFICATIONS

- *Pain in shoulder area*
  Use abbreviated movement range from arms not fully extended to hands at chin level. Slow down upward movement and pause in top position.

- *Discomfort in low back area*
  Maintain erect posture throughout exercise, with no backward lean during the pulling action.

- *Pain in wrists*
  Grip slanted sections of bar if available.

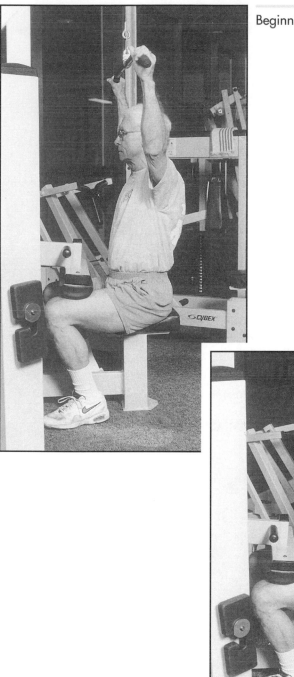

Beginning position.

Downward movement phase.

MACHINE WEIGHT-ASSISTED PULL-UP

Latissimus Dorsi, Biceps

DIRECTIONS FOR YOUR CLIENT

Beginning Position

1. Keep in mind that adding weights makes this exercise easier because they counterbalance the bodyweight.
2. Climb steps and grasp chin bar with an underhand, shoulder-width grip.
3. Place knees on platform and descend until arms are fully extended.

Upward Movement Phase

1. Pull body upward until chin is above chin bar.
2. Keep wrists straight.
3. Keep back straight.
4. Exhale throughout pulling movement.

Downward Movement Phase

1. Slowly return to starting position (until arms are fully extended).
2. Inhale throughout return movement.

POSSIBLE PROBLEMS AND RECOMMENDED MODIFICATIONS

- *Pain in shoulder area*
  Use abbreviated movement range from arms not fully extended to hands at chin level.

- *Discomfort in low back area*
  Maintain erect posture throughout exercise, with no backward lean during the pulling action.

- *Pain in wrists*
  Grip slanted sections of chin bar.

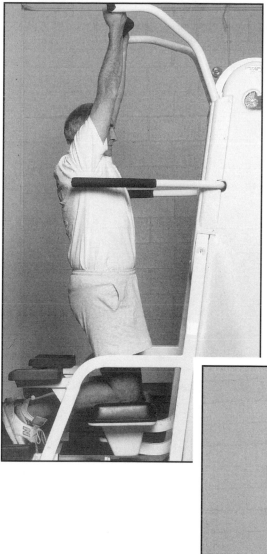

Beginning position.

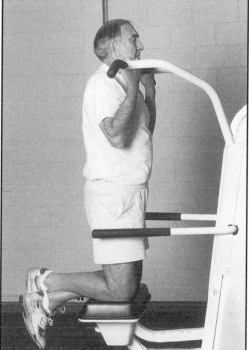

Upward movement phase.

FREE-WEIGHT DUMBBELL SEATED PRESS

Deltoids, Triceps

DIRECTIONS FOR YOUR CLIENT

Beginning Position

1. Grasp dumbbells with palms turned away, positioned at shoulder height.
2. Sit with legs straddling bench and feet in contact with floor at all times.
3. Keep head and entire back in contact with seat back.

Upward Movement Phase

1. Slowly push dumbbells upward in unison until arms are fully extended over the shoulders.
2. Exhale throughout pushing movement.

Downward Movement Phase

1. Slowly lower dumbbells in unison to shoulder level.
2. Inhale throughout lowering movement.

POSSIBLE PROBLEMS AND RECOMMENDED MODIFICATIONS

- *Pain in shoulders*
  Substitute shoulder exercise that does not require overhead movement, such as dumbbell lateral raise.

- *Discomfort in low back area*
  Contract abdominal muscles and press low back against seatback.
  NOTE: Although this exercise may be done on a flat bench, we recommend using an incline bench to provide back support and stability.

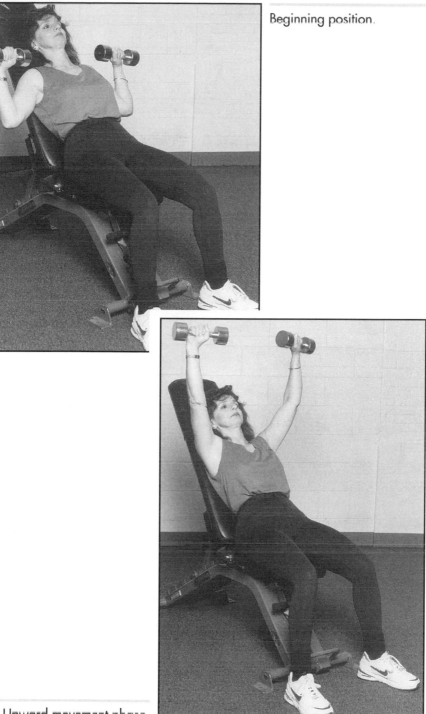

Beginning position.

Upward movement phase.

MACHINE LATERAL RAISE

Deltoids

DIRECTIONS FOR YOUR CLIENT

Beginning Position

1. Adjust seat so shoulders are in line with machine's axes of rotation.
2. Sit with head, shoulders, and back firmly against seat pad.
3. Position arms against arm pads and hands on handles, with arms close to sides.

Upward Movement Phase

1. Slowly lift arm pads upward, using arms more than hands.
2. Keep wrists straight.
3. Stop upward movement when arms are parallel to floor.
4. Exhale throughout lifting movement.

Downward Movement Phase

1. Slowly return arm pads to starting position.
2. Inhale throughout lowering movement.

POSSIBLE PROBLEMS AND RECOMMENDED MODIFICATIONS

- *Pain in shoulders*
  Stop upward movement before upper arms are parallel to floor.

- *Pain in wrists*
  Grasp handles lightly for stability, but do not use hands for lifting purposes.

- *Discomfort in low back area*
  Contract abdominal muscles to maintain flat back contact with seatback.

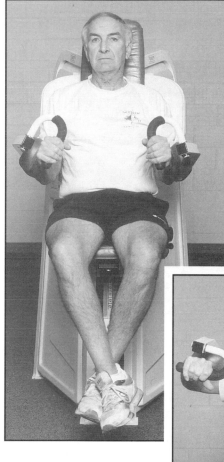

Beginning position.

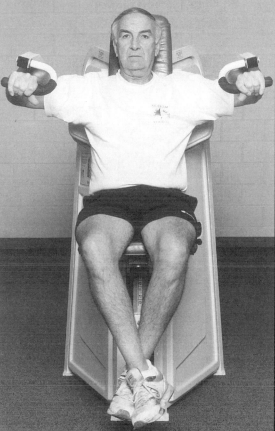

Upward movement phase.

FREE-WEIGHT DUMBBELL LATERAL RAISE

Deltoids

DIRECTIONS FOR YOUR CLIENT

Beginning Position

1. Grasp dumbbells with palms facing outer thighs and elbows slightly flexed.
2. Stand erect with feet hip-width apart.

Upward Movement Phase

1. Slowly lift dumbbells upward and sideward in unison until level with shoulders, arms parallel to floor.
2. Keep elbows slightly flexed.
3. Exhale throughout the upward movement.

Downward Movement Phase

1. Slowly lower dumbbells in unison to starting position.
2. Inhale throughout lowering movement.

POSSIBLE PROBLEMS AND RECOMMENDED MODIFICATIONS

- *Pain in shoulders*
  Stop upward movement before upper arms are parallel to floor.

- *Pain in wrists*
  Maintain neutral wrist position throughout each repetition.

- *Strain in elbows*
  Keep elbows partially flexed throughout exercise.

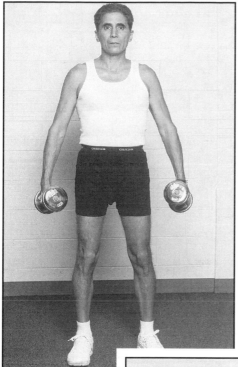

Beginning position.

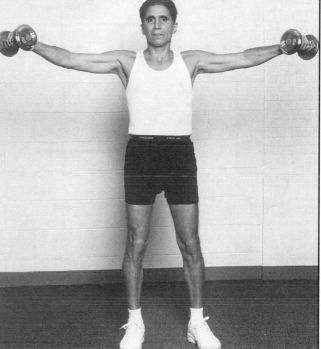

Upward movement phase.

FREE-WEIGHT DUMBBELL SHRUG

Upper Trapezius

DIRECTIONS FOR YOUR CLIENT

Beginning Position

1. Grasp dumbbells with overhand grip, arms at sides and fully extended. Keep arms straight throughout the exercise.
2. Stand erect with feet hip-width apart.

Upward Movement Phase

1. Elevate (shrug) the shoulders toward the ears as high as possible.
2. Exhale throughout shrugging movement.

Downward Movement Phase

1. Slowly lower dumbbells in unison to starting position.
2. Inhale throughout lowering movement.

POSSIBLE PROBLEMS AND RECOMMENDED MODIFICATIONS

- *Discomfort in neck area*
  Maintain neutral head position. Restrict movement range to partial shrug action.

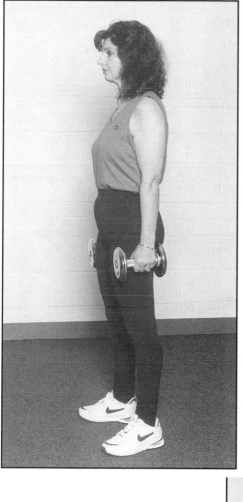

Beginning position.

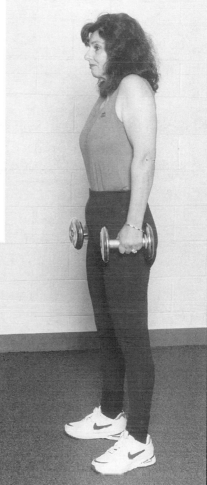

Upward movement phase.

FREE-WEIGHT BARBELL SHRUG

Upper Trapezius

DIRECTIONS FOR YOUR CLIENT

Beginning Position

1. Grasp barbell with an overhand grip, arms at sides and fully extended. Keep arms straight throughout the exercise.
2. Stand erect with feet hip-width apart.

Upward Movement Phase

1. Elevate (shrug) the shoulders toward the ears as high as possible.
2. Exhale throughout shrugging movement.

Downward Movement Phase

1. Slowly lower barbell to starting position.
2. Inhale throughout lowering movement.

POSSIBLE PROBLEMS AND RECOMMENDED MODIFICATIONS

- *Discomfort in neck area*
  Maintain neutral head position. Restrict movement range to partial shrug action.

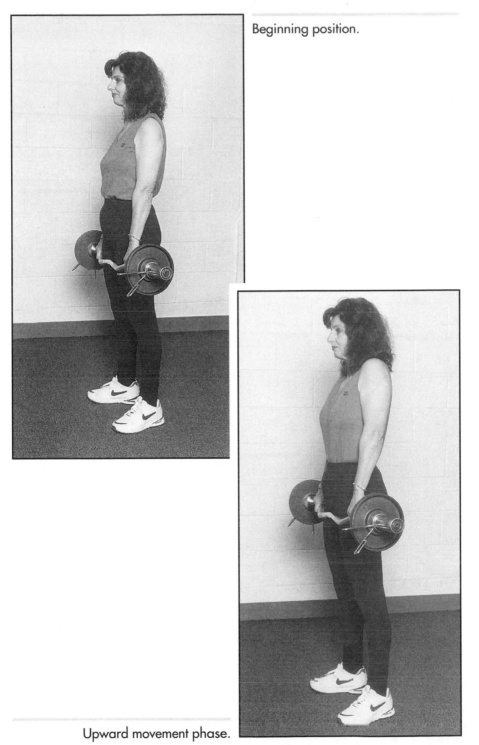

Beginning position.

Upward movement phase.

MACHINE BICEPS CURL

Biceps

DIRECTIONS FOR YOUR CLIENT

Beginning Position

1. Adjust seat so elbows are in line with machine's axis of rotation and upper arms are parallel to floor.
2. Grasp handles with underhand grip, elbows slightly flexed.
3. Sit with chest against chest pad, torso erect.

Upward Movement Phase

1. Slowly curl handles upward until elbows are fully flexed.
2. Keep wrists straight.
3. Exhale throughout lifting movement.

Downward Movement Phase

1. Slowly return handles to starting position.
2. Inhale throughout lowering movement.

POSSIBLE PROBLEMS AND RECOMMENDED MODIFICATIONS

- *Pain in elbows*
  Reposition elbows in line with machine axis of rotation. Stop about 30 degrees short of full elbow extension on lowering movements.

- *Pain in wrists*
  Maintain neutral wrist position throughout each repetition.

- *Discomfort in low back area*
  Maintain erect posture and avoid arching back.

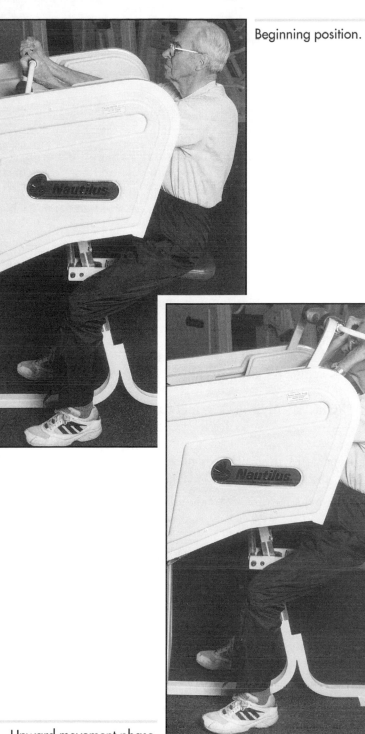

Beginning position.

Upward movement phase.

FREE-WEIGHT DUMBBELL CURL

Biceps

DIRECTIONS FOR YOUR CLIENT

Beginning Position

1. Grasp dumbbells with palms facing outer thighs, and arms straight. Ensure that upper arms remain perpendicular to floor and against sides throughout this exercise.

2. Stand erect with feet about hip-width apart and parallel to each other.

Upward Movement Phase

1. Curl dumbbells upward toward shoulders, rotating wrists until palms face the chest.

2. Exhale throughout upward movement.

Downward Movement Phase

1. Slowly lower dumbbells in unison to starting position.

2. Inhale throughout lowering movement.

POSSIBLE PROBLEMS AND RECOMMENDED MODIFICATIONS

- *Stress in shoulder area*
  Keep upper arms firmly pressed against sides throughout each repetition.

- *Discomfort in low back area*
  Maintain erect posture throughout exercise, with no backward lean during the curling action.

- *Pain in wrists*
  Keep wrists in neutral position at all times.

- *Pain in elbow area*
  Reduce wrist supination of arms during lifting movement.

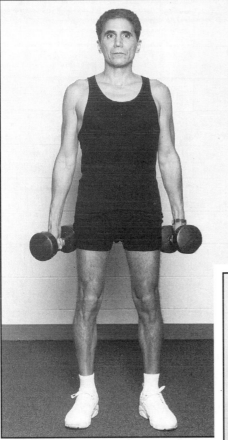

Beginning position.

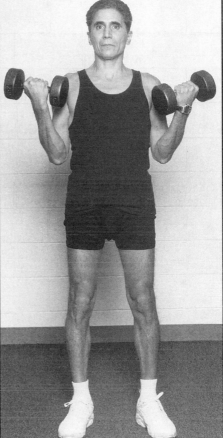

Upward movement phase.

FREE-WEIGHT DUMBBELL CONCENTRATION CURL

Biceps

DIRECTIONS FOR YOUR CLIENT

Beginning Position

1. Sit on bench, grasp dumbbell with left upper arm braced against left thigh, feet shoulder-width apart, and upper body leaning slightly forward. Upper arm should remain firmly braced against thigh throughout the exercise.
2. Begin with arm straight and palm facing away from thigh.

Upward Movement Phase

1. Curl dumbbell toward chin.
2. Exhale throughout curling movement.

Downward Movement Phase

1. Slowly lower dumbbell back to starting position.
2. Inhale throughout lowering movement.
3. Repeat from beginning position with right arm.

POSSIBLE PROBLEMS AND RECOMMENDED MODIFICATIONS

- *Stress in shoulder area*
  Use thigh to stabilize upper arm, and do not allow shoulder to be pulled downwards.

- *Discomfort in low back area*
  Use free arm for torso support and avoid excessive forward lean.

- *Pain in wrist*
  Keep wrist in neutral position at all times.

- *Pain in elbow area*
  Avoid excessive wrist supination during lifting and lowering movements.

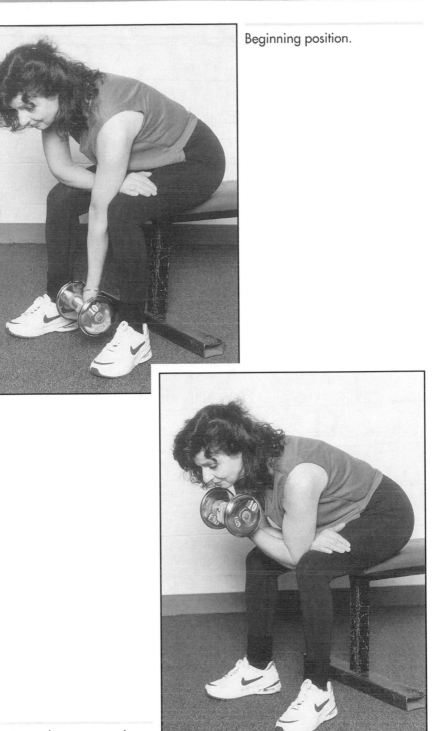

Beginning position.

Upward movement phase.

FREE-WEIGHT BARBELL CURL

Biceps

DIRECTIONS FOR YOUR CLIENT

Beginning Position

1. Grasp bar with underhand grip, with upper arms against sides. Ensure that upper arms remain perpendicular to floor and against sides throughout this exercise.
2. Stand erect with feet about hip-width apart and parallel to each other.

Upward Movement Phase

1. Slowly curl barbell upward toward shoulders.
2. Exhale throughout curling movement.

Downward Movement Phase

1. Slowly lower barbell until arms are fully extended.
2. Inhale throughout lowering movement.

POSSIBLE PROBLEMS AND RECOMMENDED MODIFICATIONS

- *Stress in shoulder area*
  Keep upper arms firmly pressed against sides throughout each repetition.

- *Discomfort in low back area*
  Maintain erect posture throughout exercise, with no backward lean during the curling action.

- *Pain in wrists*
  Keep wrists in neutral position at all times.

- *Pain in elbow area*
  Substitute dumbbell curls or angled barbell.

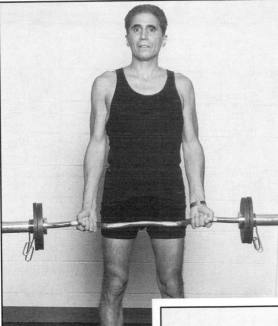

Beginning position.

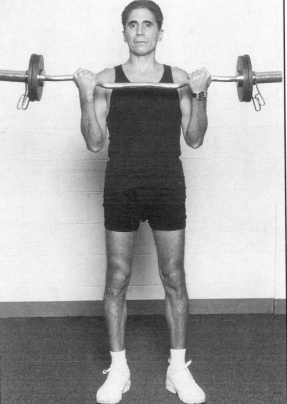

Upward movement phase.

113

MACHINE TRICEPS EXTENSION

Triceps

DIRECTIONS FOR YOUR CLIENT

Beginning Position

1. Adjust seat so elbows are in line with machine's axis of rotation and upper arms are parallel to floor.
2. Sit with back firmly against seat pad.
3. Place sides of hands against hand pads and allow pads to move close to face.

Forward Movement Phase

1. Slowly push hand pads downward until arms are fully extended.
2. Keep wrists straight.
3. Exhale throughout pushing movement.

Backward Movement Phase

1. Slowly return hand pads to the starting position.
2. Inhale throughout return movement.
3. After the final repetition, stand to remove hands from hand pads and exit seat.

POSSIBLE PROBLEMS AND RECOMMENDED MODIFICATIONS

- *Pain in elbows*
  Reposition elbows in line with machine axis of rotation. Stop about 30 degrees short of full elbow flexion on upward movement phase.

- *Pain in wrists*
  Maintain neutral wrist position throughout each repetition.

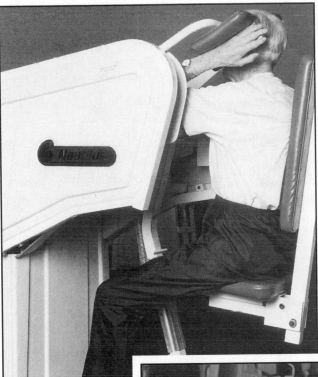

Beginning position.

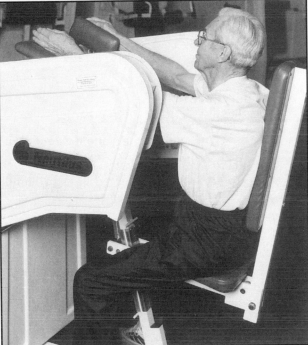

Forward movement
phase.

FREE-WEIGHT DUMBBELL OVERHEAD TRICEPS EXTENSION

Triceps

DIRECTIONS FOR YOUR CLIENT

Beginning Position

1. Grasp one dumbbell with both hands and stand erect with feet about hip-width apart.
2. Lift dumbbell upward until elbows are fully extended, directly above head. Keep upper arms perpendicular to floor throughout exercise.

Downward Movement Phase

1. Slowly lower dumbbell toward base of neck, without moving upper arms.
2. Inhale throughout lowering movement.

Upward Movement Phase

1. Lift dumbbell upward slowly until elbows are fully extended.
2. Exhale throughout lifting movement.

POSSIBLE PROBLEMS AND RECOMMENDED MODIFICATIONS

- *Pain in shoulder area*
  Substitute triceps kickback or other triceps exercise performed below shoulder level.

- *Discomfort in low back area*
  Maintain erect posture throughout exercise without excessive back arch.

- *Pain in elbows*
  Keep elbows high and near head throughout each repetition. Use abbreviated lowering movements.

- *Pain in wrists*
  Keep wrists in neutral position at all times.

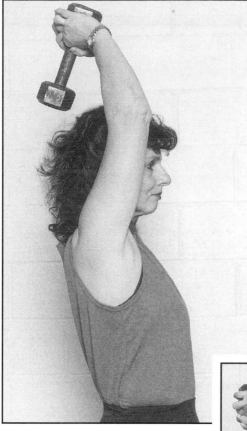

Beginning position.

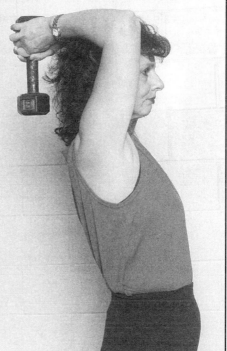

Downward movement phase.

MACHINE TRICEPS PRESS-DOWN

Triceps

DIRECTIONS FOR YOUR CLIENT

Beginning Position

1. Stand erect with feet hip-width apart and knees slightly flexed.
2. Grasp bar with overhand grip.
3. Push bar down until upper arms are perpendicular with floor and touching sides.

Downward Movement Phase

1. Push bar downward until elbows are fully extended.
2. Exhale throughout pushing movement.

Upward Movement Phase

1. Be prepared for an unexpected upward pull from the bar during the upward movement phase!
2. Return bar slowly to starting position.
3. Inhale throughout return movement.

POSSIBLE PROBLEMS AND RECOMMENDED MODIFICATIONS

- *Stress in shoulder area*
  Keep upper arms firmly pressed against sides throughout each repetition.

- *Discomfort in low back area*
  Maintain erect posture throughout exercise with no forward lean during the pressing action.

- *Pain in wrists*
  Keep wrists in neutral position at all times.

- *Pain in elbows*
  Grip press-down bar with hands about shoulder-width apart. Use angled bar to prevent excessive wrist pronation.

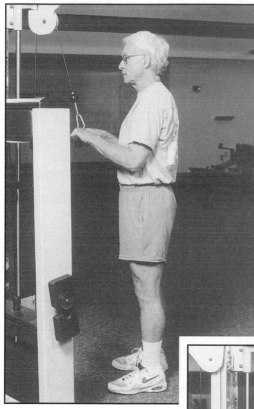

Beginning position.

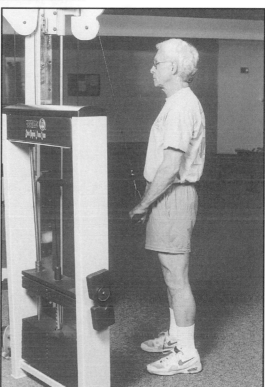

Downward movement phase.

MACHINE NECK FLEXION

Neck Flexors

DIRECTIONS FOR YOUR CLIENT

Beginning Position

1. Adjust seat so face fits comfortably against head pad, nose parallel to crossbar.
2. Adjust torso pad for erect posture.
3. Place forehead and cheeks against head pad, head angled slightly backward.
4. Grip handles.

Forward Movement Phase

1. Push head pad forward slowly until the neck is fully flexed.
2. Keep torso straight.
3. Exhale throughout forward movement.

Backward Movement Phase

1. Slowly return head pad to starting position, with head angled slightly backward.
2. Inhale throughout return movement.

POSSIBLE PROBLEMS AND RECOMMENDED MODIFICATIONS

- *Pain in neck or shoulder area*
  Reposition head against movement pad, typically helped by raising seat slightly. Maintain chest contact with support pad throughout each repetition.

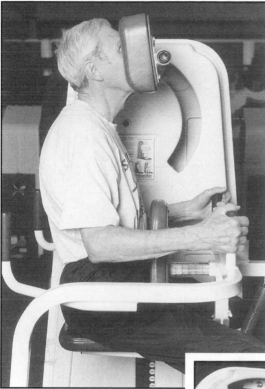

Beginning position.

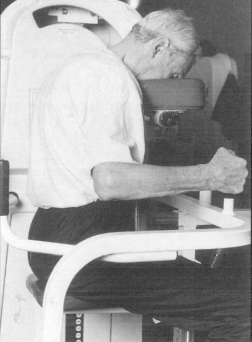

Forward movement phase.

MACHINE NECK EXTENSION

Neck Extensors

DIRECTIONS FOR YOUR CLIENT

Beginning Position

1. Adjust seat so back of head fits comfortably in head pad.
2. Adjust torso pad for an erect posture.
3. Place back of head against head pad with head angled slightly forward.
4. Grip handles.

Backward Movement Phase

1. Push head pad backward slowly until neck is comfortably extended.
2. Keep torso straight.
3. Exhale throughout backward movement.

Forward Movement Phase

1. Slowly return head pad to starting position, with head angled slightly forward.
2. Inhale throughout return movement.

POSSIBLE PROBLEMS AND RECOMMENDED MODIFICATIONS

- *Pain in neck or shoulder area*
  Reposition head against movement pad, typically helped by raising seat slightly. Maintain back contact with support pad throughout each repetition.

Note: Because the neck area is potentially difficult to train correctly and safely, we have not included neck exercises in the sample workouts in chapters 5 and 6. However, we encourage seniors to strengthen these important muscles if your clients have access to a neck machine.

Beginning position.

Backward movement phase.

Additional Machine Exercises

Although the forearm muscles are involved in all gripping exercises (e.g., holding dumbbells, barbells, chinning bars, and so on), some facilities have specially designed forearm machines that target these muscles specifically. For example, the Nautilus super-forearm machine features five separate exercises for the various forearm muscles. If your clients have access to this machine, we recommend that they regularly perform these forearm strengthening exercises.

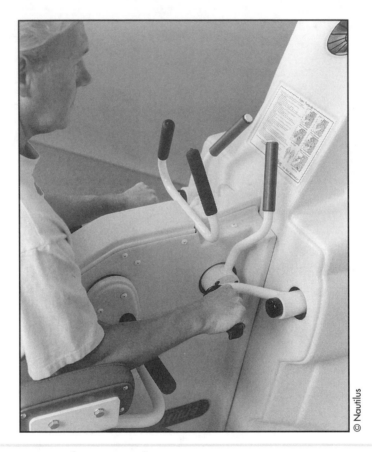

© Nautilus

Wrist pronation on forearm machine.

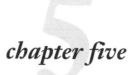

chapter five

Basic Workout Programs

Based on the exercises in chapter 4 and the training principles in chapter 3, we have designed Beginning, Intermediate, and Advanced strength-training workouts for men and women in their 50s, 60s, or 70s. The exercises use equipment typically found in fitness facilities, and the programs feature appropriate weightloads and repetitions for healthy older adults. Chapter 7 discusses alternative equipment such as elastic bands, and chapter 9 suggests modifications for older adults with various medical conditions.

We have included exercises for both machine and free-weight equipment, so you can choose a workout program that best suits your situation. If your clients have strength trained previously, or demonstrate above-average strength fitness, you can move more quickly to the Intermediate or Advanced programs presented later in this book. We strongly suggest that you follow the Beginner workout progressions with untrained clients, as well as those with prior experience but below-average strength fitness.

Recommended Weightload Assignments

To assign appropriate weightloads you must consider age, gender, previous strength training experience, current strength fitness level, and underlying medical conditions. The weightload selection tables in this chapter suggest starting weightloads for Beginner workouts and for Intermediate and Advanced clients who are performing one of these exercises for the first time.

Suggested starting weightloads for machine exercises (table 5.1 for men, table 5.2 for women) are based on data from over 200 older adults who trained on Nautilus machines (Westcott 1995). Although the suggested weightloads should result in about 8-12 repetitions, adjustments may be necessary, especially if your clients use machines made by a different manufacturer.

The starting weightloads for the free-weight exercises (table 5.3 for men, table 5.4 for women) are based upon the authors' training experiences with many older clients. These weightloads should also result in 8-12 repetitions. You will find other options for determining weightloads in the discussion of Intermediate and Advanced programs (chapter 6).

Figure 5.1 shows how to fill out Training Log 1, using information from tables 5.1 through 5.4 to assign weightloads. First determine the type of equipment to be used, and the appropriate age category; then adjust the weightloads for each exercise according to your client's strength fitness level (see the first part of chapter 8—especially table 8.1). Figure 5.1 also shows how to transfer weightload and "goal" repetition information to your clients' Training Log, and where to record dates and reps completed. (Weeks 1 and 2 of the Beginner's program are used as an example. Follow the same procedure to record information for Intermediate or Advanced workouts.) If you intend to have clients complete all three of the four-week training cycles, make six copies of the Training Log 1 before writing in training information. Copy the training log at 145% if you want an 8.5" × 11" log.

As a rule of thumb, clients with below-average strength fitness should reduce the recommended exercise weightloads in tables 5.1 through 5.4 by about 10 to 20%; those who are above average should increase the weightloads by about 10 to 20%. Reduce the resistance if a client cannot complete at least eight repetitions with good form; increase the weightload if he or she can perform more than 12 reps. Use table 5.5 to calculate changes in weightload.

Beginner Workouts

The Beginner program includes five two-week segments. It begins with five exercises that involve most of the major muscle groups, and adds new exercises every two weeks.

Beginner Workouts: Weeks 1 and 2

For *machine* equipment, the exercises for weeks 1 and 2 of the Beginner program (refer to tables 5.1 and 5.2) are performed *in this order*:

1. Leg press
2. Chest press
3. Compound row
4. Abdominal curl
5. Back extension

Table 5.1

Machine Training—Men

New exercises	Muscle group	Suggested starting weightloads (lb)		
		50-59 years	60-69 years	70-79 years
Exercises for weeks 1 and 2				
Leg press	Quadriceps Hamstrings	110.0	100.0	90.0
Chest press	Pectoralis major Anterior deltoids Triceps	50.0	45.0	40.0
Compound row	Latissimus dorsi Posterior deltoids Biceps	70.0	62.5	55.0
Abdominal curl	Rectus abdominis	55.0	50.0	45.0
Back extension	Erector spinae	55.0	50.0	45.0
Add these exercises for weeks 3 and 4				
Hip adduction	Hip adductors	65.0	60.0	55.0
Hip abduction	Hip abductors	55.0	50.0	45.0
Add these exercises for weeks 5 and 6				
Triceps extension	Triceps	45.0	40.0	35.0
Biceps curl	Biceps	45.0	40.0	35.0
Add these exercises for weeks 7 and 8				
Chest crossover	Pectoralis major	52.5	50.0	47.5
Super pullover	Latissimus dorsi	57.5	55.0	52.5
Lateral raise	Deltoids	47.5	45.0	42.5
Add these exercises for weeks 9 and 10				
Leg extension	Quadriceps	55.0	50.0	45.0
Leg curl	Hamstrings	55.0	50.0	45.0

Table 5.2

Machine Training—Women

New exercises	Muscle group	Suggested starting weightloads (lb)		
		50-59 years	60-69 years	70-79 years
Exercises for weeks 1 and 2				
Leg press	Quadriceps Hamstrings	75.0	67.5	60.0
Chest Press	Pectoralis major Anterior deltoids Triceps	32.5	30.0	27.5
Compound row	Latissimus dorsi Posterior deltoids Biceps	47.5	42.5	37.5
Abdominal curl	Rectus abdominis	37.5	35.0	32.5
Back extension	Erector spinae	37.5	35.0	32.5
Add these exercises for weeks 3 and 4				
Hip adduction	Hip adductors	47.5	45.0	42.5
Hip abduction	Hip abductors	37.5	35.0	32.5
Add these exercises for weeks 5 and 6				
Triceps extension	Triceps	25.0	22.5	20.0
Biceps curl	Biceps	25.0	22.5	20.0
Add these exercises for weeks 7 and 8				
Chest crossover	Pectoralis major	30.0	27.5	25.0
Super pullover	Latissimus dorsi	32.5	30.0	27.5
Lateral raise	Deltoids	27.5	25.0	22.5
Add these exercises for weeks 9 and 10				
Leg extension	Quadriceps	35.0	30.0	25.0
Leg curl	Hamstrings	35.0	30.0	25.0

Table 5.3

Free-Weight Training—Men

| | | Suggested starting weightloads (lb) | | |
New exercises	Muscle group	50-59 years	60-69 years	70-79 years
Exercises for weeks 1 and 2				
Dumbbell squat	Quadriceps Hamstrings	25.0	20.0	15.0
Dumbbell bench press	Pectoralis major Anterior deltoids Triceps	25.0	20.0	15.0
Dumbbell one-arm row	Latissimus dorsi Posterior deltoids Biceps	25.0	20.0	15.0
Dumbbell seated press	Deltoids Triceps	20.0	15.0	10.0
Trunk curl	Rectus abdominis	20 reps	15 reps	10 reps
Add these exercises for weeks 3 and 4				
Dumbbell biceps curl	Biceps	15.0	12.5	10.0
Dumbbell overhead triceps extension	Triceps	15.0	12.5	10.0
Add these exercises for weeks 5 and 6				
Dumbbell shrug	Upper trapezius	25.0	20.0	15.0
Dumbbell heel raise	Gastrocnemius/soleus	25.0	20.0	15.0
Add these exercises for weeks 7 and 8				
Dumbbell chest fly	Pectoralis major	15.0	12.5	10.0
Add these exercises for weeks 9 and 10				
Lat pulldown	Latissimus dorsi Biceps	60.0	50.0	40.0
Triceps press-down	Triceps	35.0	30.0	25.0

Table 5.4

		Suggested starting weightloads (lb)		
New exercises	**Muscle group**	**50-59 years**	**60-69 years**	**70-79 years**
Exercises for weeks 1 and 2				
Dumbbell squat	Quadriceps Hamstrings	15.0	12.5	10.0
Dumbbell bench press	Pectoralis major Anterior deltoids Triceps	12.5	10.0	7.5
Dumbbell one-arm row	Latissimus dorsi Posterior deltoids Biceps	12.5	10.0	7.5
Dumbbell seated press	Deltoids Triceps	12.5	10.0	7.5
Trunk curl	Rectus abdominis	15 reps	10 reps	5 reps
Add these exercises for weeks 3 and 4				
Dumbbell biceps curl	Biceps	10.0	7.5	5.0
Dumbbell overhead triceps extension	Triceps	7.5	5.0	2.5
Add these exercises for weeks 5 and 6				
Dumbbell shrug	Upper trapezius	15.0	12.5	10.0
Dumbbell heel raise	Gastrocnemius/soleus	15.0	12.5	10.0
Add these exercises for weeks 7 and 8				
Dumbbell chest fly	Pectoralis major	10.0	7.5	5.0
Add these exercises for weeks 9 and 10				
Lat pulldown	Latissimus dorsi Biceps	40.0	35.0	30.0
Triceps press-down	Triceps	25.0	20.0	15.0

Free-Weight Training—Women

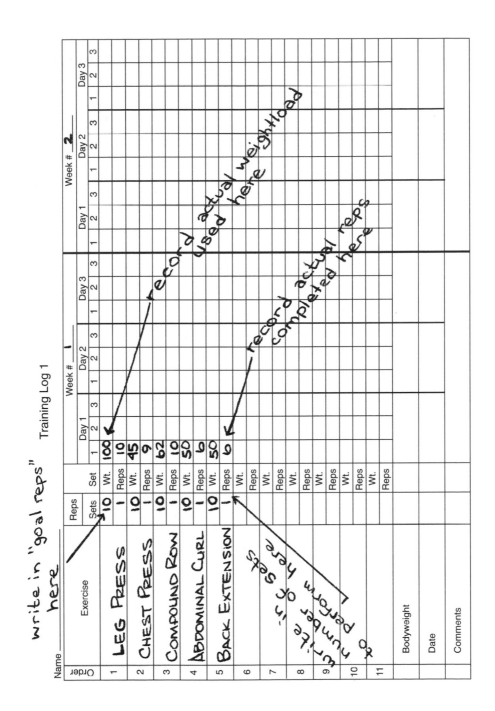

Figure 5.1 How to record workout information in the training log.

Table 5.5

Load Adjustment Guidelines for Repetitions Completed		
Reps	Below goal subtract (lb)	Above goal add (lb)
1	2.5	2.5
2	5.0	5.0
3	7.5	7.5
4	10.0	10.0
5	12.5	12.5
6	15.0	15.0

In the left hand column identify the number of reps that your client performed below or above the "Goal Reps" listed in the training log for a particular exercise. Subtract the weight listed in the "Below Goal" column from the current weightload if your client performed too few reps. Add the weight in the "Above Goal" column if your client performed too many reps.

For *free-weight* equipment, exercises for weeks 1 and 2 (tables 5.3 and 5.4) are performed *in this order*:

1. Dumbbell squat
2. Dumbbell bench press
3. Dumbbell one-arm row
4. Dumbbell seated press
5. Trunk curl

Copy Training Log 1 for your clients' use (copy at 145% for an 8.5" × 11" log). If you have questions about how to fill out the Training Log, study figure 5.1. Be sure that your clients perform these exercises in the order in which they are listed. As you add exercises to Beginners' workouts in weeks 3, 5, 7, and 9, refer to tables 5.1 through 5.4 for appropriate weightload assignments. Instruct beginning clients to perform 8-12 repetitions in all exercises except the free-weight trunk curl, in which they should perform 15-30 repetitions. In all other exercises, as soon as your client is able to perform 12 repetitions with good form during two consecutive workouts, increase the weightload by 1.25 to 2.5 pounds.

Beginner Workouts: Weeks 3 and 4

At this point your clients are strengthening most of their major muscle groups, and the exercise movement patterns should be second nature. Because many older adults are concerned about hip function, we suggest that you add two exercises to the machine training program if the machines are available—the hip adduction machine for the hip adductor muscles and the hip abduction machine for the hip abductor muscles. Insert these exercises between the leg press and the chest press.

For a free-weight program, the squat exercise that is already included is an excellent hip strengthener, so you need not add other lower body exercises at this time. Instead, complement the basic workout with dumbbell curls for the biceps muscles and dumbbell overhead triceps extension for the triceps muscles. These two new exercises should be done after the dumbbell press and before the trunk curls.

For a *machine* exercise program, then, the exercises during weeks 3 and 4 (again, refer to tables 5.1 and 5.2) are performed *in this order*:

1. Leg press
2. Hip adductor
3. Hip abductor
4. Chest press
5. Compound row
6. Abdominal curl
7. Back extension

For a *free-weight* program, the exercises during weeks 3 and 4 are performed *in this order*:

1. Dumbbell squat
2. Dumbbell bench press
3. Dumbbell one-arm row
4. Dumbbell seated press
5. Dumbbell biceps curl
6. Dumbbell overhead triceps extension
7. Trunk curl

Record either the machine or free-weight exercises, in the order presented, onto a Training Log (see page 207) and label this Training Log "Weeks 3 and 4".

Beginner Workouts: Weeks 5 and 6

The machine training program involves three exercises for the legs, two for the trunk, and two for the upper body. Although the arms are involved in both the chest press and compound row exercises, triceps extensions and biceps curls will train these muscles more directly. The triceps extension machine targets the triceps muscles, and the biceps curl machine targets the biceps muscles. Add these two exercises between the compound row and abdominal curl exercises.

If your client is training with free weights, add the dumbbell shrug for the upper trapezius and the dumbbell heel raise for the gastrocnemius/soleus muscles. These new exercises should follow all the other exercises.

The *machine* exercise program during weeks 5 and 6, then, comprises the following exercises to be performed *in this order*:

1. Leg press
2. Hip adductor
3. Hip abductor
4. Chest press
5. Compound row
6. Triceps extension
7. Biceps curl
8. Abdominal curl
9. Back extension

For weeks 5 and 6 of a *free-weight* program, your clients should perform the following exercises *in this order*:

1. Dumbbell squat
2. Dumbbell bench press
3. Dumbbell one-arm row
4. Dumbbell seated press
5. Dumbbell biceps curl
6. Dumbbell overhead triceps extension
7. Trunk curl
8. Dumbbell shrug
9. Dumbbell heel raise

Record either the machine or free-weight exercises, in the order presented, onto a Training Log (see page 207) and label this Training Log "Weeks 5 and 6".

Beginner Workouts: Weeks 7 and 8

After six weeks of regular strength training, your clients should have more muscle and less fat, and should feel stronger than when they entered the program. At this point you may want to spend a little time explaining some of the adaptations that the muscles are making as a result of regular strength training (chapter 1, page 3). If your client is using machines, replace the chest press and compound row with three exercises that better target the chest, upper back, and shoulder muscles: the chest crossover for the pectoralis major, super pullover for latissimus dorsi, and lateral raise for the middle deltoids.

If your client is using free weights, complement the dumbbell bench press exercise with the dumbbell chest fly exercise to emphasize chest development. This exercise better isolates the pectoralis major muscle and should be performed after the dumbbell bench press.

Thus, in a *machine* exercise program, the exercises for weeks 7 and 8 are performed *in this order*:

1. Leg press
2. Hip adductor
3. Hip abductor
4. Chest crossover
5. Super pullover
6. Lateral raise
7. Triceps extension
8. Biceps curl
9. Abdominal curl
10. Back extension

In a *free-weight* exercise program, the exercises for weeks 7 and 8 are performed *in this order*:

1. Dumbbell squat
2. Dumbbell bench press
3. Dumbbell chest fly
4. Dumbbell one-arm row
5. Dumbbell seated press
6. Dumbbell biceps curl
7. Dumbbell overhead triceps extension
8. Trunk curl
9. Dumbbell shrug
10. Dumbbell heel raise

Record either the machine or free-weight exercises in the order presented onto a Training Log (see page 207) and label this Training Log "Weeks 7 and 8".

Beginner Workouts: Weeks 9 and 10

Just as you changed the upper body machine exercises to better target the chest, upper back, and shoulder muscles, you can now better isolate your clients' leg muscles. Replace the leg press with the leg extension and leg curl exercises. The leg extension addresses the quadriceps muscles, and the leg curl addresses the hamstrings muscles.

If clients following a free-weight program have access to a pulley apparatus on which they can perform lat pulldowns and triceps press-downs, consider substituting these exercises for the dumbbell one-arm row and the dumbbell overhead triceps extension. The lat pulldown works the latissimus dorsi and biceps muscles, and the triceps press-down works the triceps muscles. The pulley exercises provide excellent training for these muscle groups and add variety to the workout program. If you do not have access to this equipment, continue doing the dumbbell one-arm row and dumbbell overhead triceps extension exercises.

For a *machine* exercise program in weeks 9 and 10, the exercises are performed *in this order:*

1. Leg extension
2. Leg curl
3. Hip adductor
4. Hip abductor
5. Chest crossover
6. Super pullover
7. Lateral raise
8. Triceps extension
9. Biceps curl
10. Abdominal curl
11. Back extension

For a *free-weight* exercise program, the exercises for weeks 9 and 10 are performed *in this order:*

1. Dumbbell squat
2. Dumbbell bench press
3. Dumbbell chest fly
4. Lat pulldown
5. Dumbbell seated press
6. Dumbbell biceps curl
7. Triceps press-down
8. Trunk curl
9. Dumbbell shrug
10. Dumbbell heel raise

Record either the machine or free-weight exercises in the order presented onto a Training Log (see page 207), and label this Training Log "Weeks 9 and 10".

What Next?

Your clients have now completed 10 weeks of regular strength training exercises, working all of their major muscle groups productively and progressively. The results should be obvious. At this point you have many options for continuing or changing their strength training program. For example, you can alternate different exercises for the target muscles, thereby increasing the training variety and the developmental stimulus. If you want, you can also combine machine and free-weight training exercises.

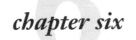

chapter six

Intermediate and Advanced Workout Programs

If your clients have the time and desire to expand their strength training workouts, they may perform more sets of each exercise or additional exercises for each major muscle group. You can also use different training protocols to emphasize larger muscle size, greater muscle strength, or more muscle endurance. This chapter will help you design such programs.

Intermediate Workouts

The 10-week Beginner training program provided a sensible progression of strength exercises and starting weightloads for completing 8-12 repetitions. The systematic integration of these exercises enabled your clients to master the performance techniques and to adapt physiologically to the training program. As your clients near the end of the 10-week program, they may ask what they should do next. You may want them to continue their current workouts because they have experienced excellent improvements in muscle strength and body composition. If so, be sure to vary the exercises periodically, and progressively increase the training resistance as your clients become stronger.

If Your Clients Decide to Take the Challenge

You may also decide to introduce a capable client to more challenging workouts. If so, this can be an exciting time! Their muscle strength should be sufficient to handle heavier loads, and their muscle endurance should be adequate to complete longer and more demanding workouts. Obviously, the purpose of more comprehensive workouts is to produce even greater strength gains and muscle development. Just be sensible in the approach you take. Always keep your clients' ability levels in mind, reinforce the importance of proper form, and add exercises, sets, and resistance gradually.

For more advanced strength training, you can choose from three Intermediate programs included in this chapter. Each one is designed to further develop muscle size, muscle strength, or muscle endurance.

Once you have decided which outcome best meets your clients' needs, refer to the appropriate sample training program. These workouts offer the option of using free weights or machines, or a combination of both. Just be sure to apply the training principles in chapter 3 and the training procedures and teaching strategies in chapter 4. Make six more copies of the Training Log 1 in the appendix for recording the results (reminder: enlarge at 145% to get 8.5" × 11" forms).

The training options presented here build on the 10-week program of exercises in the Beginner workouts. To reduce the chance of setbacks caused by doing too much too soon, each program starts with a four-week transition period. Following the transition period is a less intense training week followed by a four-week program of greater intensity. A less intense week occurs again and is followed by another four-week program of more intense training time. The four-week programs described here are referred to as training cycles. Each training cycle presents workouts that are more intense than the preceding one.

As the workouts become more demanding, the time required to complete them increases. To help you schedule your clients' training sessions, we have listed the approximate amount of time necessary for completing workouts at the end of each program. We have kept the workouts as brief as possible without sacrificing effectiveness. If clients can devote only limited time to exercise, use the transition period workouts (weeks 1 through 4) for their standard training program because these require less time than the more comprehensive programs (weeks 6-9 and 11-14).

The following directions should help you adapt the 10-week Beginner program to the more intense training cycles presented next. Before deciding which workouts you will have your clients follow, consider the equipment requirements for the selected program. Also note that you must spot the barbell squat, heel raise, and bench press exercises if your clients use free-weight equipment.

Whichever program you choose for your clients, be sure to do the following:

- Record exercises, weightloads, and goal reps onto Training Log 1 (page 207).
- Teach clients how to record dates and the number of repetitions completed for each workout (suggestion: use figure 5.1).
- Remind clients to perform exercises in the order in which they are listed.
- Encourage clients to perform the number of repetitions indicated, expecting that the number of reps they complete in the second and third sets will be fewer than those in the preceding set.
- When clients are performing more than one set of an exercise, and exceed the specified number of reps in the final set on two successive workouts, increase the weightload as indicated in table 5.5.
- If clients cannot complete the desired number of repetitions, decrease the weightloads as recommended in table 5.5.
- If your clients have been training with dumbbells and you change to barbell exercises, you will need to increase their weightloads. A good rule of thumb is to *double* the dumbbell weight (weight of one dumbbell) you are using in the same exercise.
- If you decide to add additional exercises or perform more sets, and especially if you decide to do both, consider a four-day-a-week program described in the Advanced programs section of this chapter.

Workouts That Emphasize Muscle Size

Modify the 10-week Beginner program (chapter 5) in the following ways to emphasize muscle size improvements:

- Prescribe 8-12 repetitions per exercise, which should require increased weightloads (see tables 6.1a and b). Adding about 5 pounds to the exercises in the Beginner program should reduce the number of repetitions to the lower end of the 8-12 rep range. The 10 weeks of training leading up to these workouts should have prepared the muscles for these heavier weightloads. However, if you are not confident about increasing your clients' weightloads by 5 pounds at a time, you may add 2.5 pounds in week 1 and another 2.5 pounds in week 2.
- In the free-weight training program, you have the option of substituting barbell exercises; we have also added a new biceps exercise, the dumbbell concentration curl. Remember, if your client wants to use barbells, double the weight being used in the dumbbell curl. We have added the weight-assisted pull-up and bar dip exercises to the machine training program—try using 40% of bodyweight for male clients and 60% for

female clients. The weightload in these exercises is used to counterbalance body weight, so adding weight actually makes them easier to perform. Again, refer to table 5.5 if load adjustments are needed. You may want to add different exercises if your client expresses a desire to emphasize a muscle area other than the arms.

- Increase the number of sets in certain exercises to two for the first four weeks, then three or four in the last four weeks. In other exercises, the number of sets increases to two during the second four-week cycle and remains at two in the third cycle (see tables 6.1a and b).

- Although rest periods should remain at one minute, increase them to one and one-half or two minutes if you feel a client requires more complete recovery.

- Set a goal of 30 reps in both sets of the trunk curl exercises during weeks 1-4; 35 reps in weeks 6-9; and 40 reps in weeks 11-14.

Table 6.1a

Intermediate Machine Program for Muscle Size Development (Three Nonconsecutive Days)

| | | | Training Cycles | | |
| | | Goal | Weeks 1-4 | Weeks 6-9 | Weeks 11-14 |
Order	Exercise	Reps	Sets	Sets	Sets
1	Leg extension	8-12	2	3	3
2	Leg curl	8-12	2	3	3
3	Chest crossover	8-12	2	2	3
4	Chest press	8-12	2	3	3
5	Compound row	8-12	2	2	3
6	Lateral raise	8-12	1	2	2
7	Triceps extension	8-12	2	3	3
8	Biceps curl	8-12	2	3	3
9	Weight-assisted bar dips	8-12	1	2	2
10	Weight-assisted pull-ups	8-12	1	2	2
11	Back extension	8-12	1	2	2
12	Abdominal curl	8-12	1	2	2
Estimated time requirements (min)			42	60	64

Note: Weeks 4, 9, and 14 should be followed with a less intense week of training in which weightloads are reduced by 10 pounds and only one set of each exercise is performed.

- After each training cycle, your clients should benefit from a week of less intense training. This break from the mental "repetitiveness" of the training program will also allow muscles to gain some needed rest, rebuild tissue, and get stronger. At this point, have them perform only *one* set of 8-12 reps of each exercise except the trunk curl. Keep the reps in the trunk curl the same. After week 15, resume the workout program performed in weeks 1 and 2 (tables 6.1a or b), adjusting loads appropriately as indicated in table 5.5. Thereafter, plan a less intense week of training after the fourth week of every training cycle. This protocol (including a week of less intense training) is also important to follow if you intend to have clients follow one of the more advanced programs at the end of this chapter.

Workouts That Emphasize Strength Development

To emphasize strength building, modify the 10-week Beginner program (chapter 5) in the following ways:

Table 6.1b

Intermediate Free-Weight Program for Muscle Size Development (Three Nonconsecutive Days)

| | | | Training Cycles | | |
| | | Goal | Weeks 1-4 | Weeks 6-9 | Weeks 11-14 |
Order	Exercise	Reps	Sets	Sets	Sets
1	Dumbbell or barbell squat	8-12	2	3	3
2	Dumbbell or barbell bench press	8-12	2	3	3
3	Dumbbell chest fly	8-12	1	2	2
4	Dumbbell one-arm row	8-12	2	2	2
5	Dumbbell lateral raise	8-12	1	2	2
6	Dumbbell or barbell curl	8-12	2	3	3
7	Dumbbell concentration curl	8-12	1	2	2
8	Dumbbell overhead triceps extension	8-12	1	2	2
9	Barbell shrug	8-12	1	2	2
10	Trunk curl	30-45	1	2	2
Estimated time requirements (min)			42	60	63

Note: Weeks 4, 9, and 14 should be followed with a less intense week of training in which weightloads are reduced by 10 pounds and only one set of each exercise is performed.

- In the exercises marked with an asterisk (see tables 6.2a and 6.2b), gradually increase the weightload so that the number of repetitions decreases—from 8-12 down to 6-8—during weeks 1 through 2. To put your clients in the 6-8 repetition range for these exercises, add about 10 pounds to the present weightloads. If adding 10 pounds fails to achieve the rep range of 6-8, make appropriate weightload adjustments using table 5.5 as a guide. However, if you are not confident about increasing a client's weightloads by 10 pounds all at once, add 2.5 pounds in week 1 and another 2.5 pounds in week 2; then add 5 more pounds during week 3. Whenever your client completes 2 or more repetitions beyond the goal in the final set during two consecutive workouts, increase the weightload by 2.5 pounds.

- For exercises without an asterisk, instruct clients to perform 12 repetitions, again referring to table 5.5 if load adjustments are needed. When clients are able to complete 14 or more repetitions in the last exercise set on two consecutive occasions, increase the weightload by 2.5 pounds.

Table 6.2a

Intermediate Machine Program for Strength Development (Three Nonconsecutive Days)

| | | | Training Cycles | | |
| | | Goal | Weeks 1-4 | Weeks 6-9 | Weeks 11-14 |
Order	Exercise	Reps	Sets	Sets	Sets
1	*Leg press	6-8	1	2	3
2	Heel raise	12	2	2	2
3	*Chest crossover	6-8	1	2	3
4	*Compound row	6-8	1	2	3
5	Lateral raise	12	2	2	2
6	Triceps extension	12	2	2	2
7	Biceps curl	12	2	2	2
8	Back extension	12	2	2	2
9	Abdominal curl	12	2	2	2
Estimated time requirements (min)			56	75	80

*In the exercises marked with an asterisk, gradually increase weightloads which will reduce the number of repetitions—from 8-12 down to 6-8—during weeks 1 through 2.

Note: Weeks 4, 9, and 14 should be followed with a less intense week of training in which weightloads are reduced by 10 pounds and only one set of each exercise is performed.

- For exercises in the 6-8 rep range, increase the number of sets from one to two during the second four-week cycle, and to three during the last four-week cycle. In the 12-rep exercises, the number of sets increases to two during the first four-week cycle and remains at two throughout the second and third cycles (see tables 6.2a and b).
- Increase the length of the rest periods between sets to three minutes. Longer rest periods allow more time for the muscles to recover, enabling the use of relatively heavy weightloads in succeeding sets.
- After each training cycle, your clients will benefit from a week of less intense training. Have them perform only one set of each exercise, with the same number of reps (6-8 or 8-12) listed for each exercise. After week 15, they may resume the workout they were doing in weeks 1 and 2, with appropriate weightload adjustments as indicated in table 5.5. Thereafter, plan a less intense week of training after the fourth week of every training cycle. This procedure is also recommended if your clients follow one of the more advanced programs at the end of this chapter.

Table 6.2b

Intermediate Free-Weight Program for Strength Development (Three Nonconsecutive Days)

| | | | Training Cycles | | |
| | | | Weeks 1-4 | Weeks 6-9 | Weeks 11-14 |
Order	Exercise	Reps	Sets	Sets	Sets
1	*Dumbbell or barbell squat	6-8	1	2	3
2	Dumbbell or barbell heel raise	12	2	2	2
3	*Dumbbell or barbell bench press	6-8	1	2	3
4	*Dumbbell one-arm row	6-8	1	2	3
5	Dumbbell lateral raise	12	1	3	3
6	Dumbbell or barbell curl	12	2	2	2
7	Dumbbell overhead triceps extension	12	2	2	2
8	Trunk curl	30	2	2	2
Estimated time requirements (min)			45	63	67

*In the exercises marked with an asterisk, gradually increase weightloads which will reduce the number of repetitions—from 8-12 down to 6-8—during weeks 1 through 2.

Note: Weeks 4, 9, and 14 should be followed with a less intense week of training in which weightloads are reduced by 10 pounds and only one set of each exercise is performed.

Workouts That Emphasize Muscle Endurance

To enhance muscle endurance, modify the Beginner 10-week training program as follows:

- Increase the number of repetitions in these workouts to 12 (see tables 6.3a and 6.3b).
- Progressively increase your clients' reps to 15 while using the same weightload. Once they complete 17 or more repetitions in the last set on two consecutive occasions, increase the load by 2.5 pounds.
- Increase the number of sets in certain exercises to two in the first four-week cycle, then to three during the last four-week cycle. In other exercises, increase the number of sets to two for both the second and third four-week cycles (see tables 6.3a and b).
- Rest periods of one minute remain the same, even when multiple sets are performed.

Table 6.3a

Intermediate Machine Program for Muscle Endurance Development (Three Nonconsecutive Days)

| | | | Training Cycles | | |
| | | Goal | Weeks 1-4 | Weeks 6-9 | Weeks 11-14 |
Order	Exercise	Reps	Sets	Sets	Sets
1	Leg extension	12-15	2	2	3
2	Leg curl	12-15	2	2	3
3	Hip abduction	12-15	1	2	2
4	Hip adduction	12-15	1	2	2
5	Chest crossover	12-15	2	2	3
6	Super pullover	12-15	2	2	3
7	Lateral raise	12-15	2	2	3
8	Triceps extension	12-15	2	2	3
9	Biceps curl	12-15	2	2	3
10	Rotary torso	12-15	1	2	2
Estimated time requirements (min)			40	55	65

Note: Weeks 4, 9, and 14 should be followed with a less intense week of training in which weightloads are reduced by 10 pounds and only one set of each exercise is performed.

- Encourage your clients to perform 30 reps in both sets of the trunk curl during weeks 1-4; 35 reps in weeks 6-9; and 40 reps in weeks 11-14.
- After each training cycle, your clients will benefit from a week of less intense training for the reasons mentioned on page 141. Prescribe only one set of 15 reps in each exercise. After week 15, your clients should resume the workouts they were performing in weeks 1 and 2 (table 6.3a or 6.3b), making appropriate load adjustments as indicated in table 5.5. Thereafter, plan a less intense week of training after the fourth week of every training cycle. Also, if you intend to have clients perform one of the more intense training programs at the end of this chapter, prescribe a less intense week of training just prior to initiating the more advanced program.

If body reproportioning is the primary goal of a client, it is likely that he or she has too much fat, too little muscle, or both. Consider one or all of these actions to help achieve better body composition:

Table 6.3b

Intermediate Free-Weight Program for Muscle Endurance Development (Three Nonconsecutive Days)

| | | | Training Cycles | | |
| | | Goal | Weeks 1-4 | Weeks 6-9 | Weeks 11-14 |
Order	Exercise	Reps	Sets	Sets	Sets
1	Dumbbell or barbell squat	12-15	2	2	3
2	Dumbbell or barbell heel raise	12-15	1	2	2
3	Dumbbell or barbell bench press	12-15	2	2	3
4	Dumbbell chest fly	12-15	1	2	2
5	Dumbbell one-arm row	12-15	2	2	3
6	Dumbbell seated press	12-15	2	2	3
7	Dumbbell or barbell biceps curl	12-15	2	2	3
8	Dumbbell overhead triceps extension	12-15	2	2	3
9	Barbell shrug	12-15	1	2	2
10	Trunk curl	30-40	2	2	2
Estimated time requirements (min)			44	54	65

Note. Weeks 4, 9, and 14 should be followed with a less intense week of training in which weightloads are reduced by 10 pounds and only one set of each exercise is performed.

- Follow the muscle size program described earlier in this chapter to increase muscle mass.
- Encourage clients to select foods more carefully, and emphasize the importance of reducing fat and calorie intake. See chapter 10 for relevant information.
- Design an aerobic (endurance) program to help burn more calories. For additional guidance in this area, refer to the texts *Fitness Weight Training* by Baechle and Earle (1995) and *Building Strength and Stamina* by Westcott (1996).

Recording Workout Information in the Training Logs

Once you have decided which program (muscle size, muscle strength, or muscle endurance) and which type of equipment (machines, free-weights) your client will be following, the next step is to record his training information onto the appropriate Training Log. Make six copies of Training Log 1 if you plan to follow all three four-week training cycles (reminder: enlarge at 145% for 8.5" × 11" forms). If necessary, refer to figure 5.1 for a review of how to transfer information regarding "goal reps," number of sets to perform, and weightloads. This figure also shows where to record training dates, the number of reps completed, and comments about the workout.

Advanced Workouts

The Advanced training workouts, like the Intermediate, permit you to emphasize muscle size, strength, or endurance. Each program is four weeks in length, except the muscular endurance program which has two and eight week cycles. Presented first are those workouts that emphasize muscle size, followed by programs designed to enhance muscle strength, then muscle endurance. Unlike the Intermediate workouts, the muscle size and strength workouts involve what is referred to as the split system of training. This Advanced training method splits up the exercises according to "body parts," working some muscles two days a week and other muscles on two different days. This type of training protocol enables you to spread your clients' exercises over four days instead of three, reducing the amount of time needed to complete each workout. This arrangement also offers the opportunity to add more exercises and sets while keeping each workout length reasonable. Because your clients can perform a wider variety of exercises each session, they are able to emphasize muscle size and strength development in specific muscle groups. Examples of such an arrangement are presented later.

The disadvantage of the split training approach is that your clients must add an extra training day in their week.

Split training programs require four workouts a week. Choose a program that best fits your client's schedule. Each of the following protocols uses two workouts each for the upper and lower body, while providing sufficient rest days between weight training days:

1. Monday, Thursday—upper body; Tuesdays, Fridays—lower body.
2. Sundays, Wednesdays—upper body; Mondays, Thursdays—lower body.
3. Tuesdays, Fridays—upper body; Wednesdays, Saturdays—lower body.

If your client will be using the Advanced muscle size or the Advanced strength development programs, make four copies of Training Log 2.

Training Days: Muscle Endurance

As explained in chapter 3, your clients should not work the same muscle groups on two consecutive days, nor allow three days to go by between training sessions. For muscle endurance workouts, therefore, we suggest that you have clients follow a Monday/Wednesday/Friday or a Tuesday/Thursday/Saturday schedule.

Use Training Log 1 in the appendix for the Advanced muscle endurance program.

Advanced Muscle Size Development Programs

The four-week Advanced muscle size program shown in table 6.4 includes four workouts each week—two training days for the upper body, two for the lower body. The exercises listed in the upper body workouts include two each for the chest and back, and one each for the shoulders, biceps, and triceps. The lower body exercises include two for the combined thigh muscles and one each for the hamstrings, quadriceps, calves, and abdominal muscles.

Have clients perform 10-12 reps of the seven upper- and six lower-body exercises listed. During the fifth week reduce your clients' weightloads by 10 pounds, and have them perform only one set of each exercise during each workout. The reduced weightload and number of sets will permit the muscles to recover and build to higher strength levels. For weeks six through nine, have clients increase the number of sets in the exercises as shown in table 6.5, and make needed weightload increases as indicated in table 5.5. For week ten, have clients follow the directions given for week five. If they want to engage in more intense split training workouts, and if you feel it would be safe for them to do so, refer to the book *Fitness Weight Training* by Baechle and Earle.

Table 6.4

Advanced Muscle Size Program Weeks 1-4 (First Cycle)					
Order	Muscle group	Reps	Sets	Free-weight	Machine
Upper body exercises: 28 min					
1	Chest	10-12	2	Bench press	Chest press
2	Chest	10-12	2	Dumbbell fly	Chest crossover
3	Back	10-12	2	Dumbbell row	Compound row
4	Shoulder	10-12	2	Standing dumbbell press	Shoulder press
5	Back	10-12	2	Lat pulldown	Pulldown or pullover
6	Triceps	10-12	2	Dumbbell triceps extension	Triceps extension
7	Biceps	10-12	2	Biceps curl	Biceps curl
Lower body exercises: 22 min					
1	Thigh	10-12	2	Squat	Double leg press
2	Thigh	10-12	2	Lunge	Single leg press
3	Hamstrings	10-12	2	Leg curl	Leg curl
4	Quadriceps	10-12	2	Leg extension	Leg extension
5	Calf	10-12	2	Standing heel raise	Heel raise
6	Abdomen	30	2	Trunk curl	
		10-12	2		Abdominal curl

Note: Week 4 should be followed with a less intense week of training in which weightloads are reduced by 10 pounds and only one set of each exercise is performed.

Advanced Strength Training Programs

The four-week Advanced muscle strength program described in table 6.6 includes two upper and two lower body workouts each week. Your clients will perform two to three sets of 8-10 reps in most exercises during the first two weeks, then 6-8 reps during weeks three and four in exercises marked with an asterisk. The exercises are similar to those in the muscle size program. Reduce the weightload by 10 pounds in these exercises during the fifth week, and have clients perform only one set each training day. The lighter effort during the

Table 6.5

Advanced Muscle Size Program
Weeks 6-9 (Second Cycle)

Order	Muscle group	Reps	Sets	Free-weight	Machine
			Upper body exercises: 34 min		
1	Chest	10-12	3	Bench press	Chest press
2	Chest	10-12	2	Dumbbell fly	Chest crossover
3	Back	10-12	2	Dumbbell row	Compound row
4	Shoulder	10-12	3	Standing lateral raise	Shoulder press
5	Back	10-12	2	Lat pulldown	Pulldown or pullover
6	Triceps	10-12	2	Dumbbell triceps extension	Triceps extension
7	Biceps	10-12	3	Biceps curl	Biceps curl
			Lower body exercises: 37 min		
1	Thigh	10-12	3	Squat	Double leg press
2	Thigh	10-12	2	Lunge	Single leg press
3	Hamstrings	10-12	2	Leg curl	Leg curl
4	Quadriceps	10-12	2	Leg extension	Leg extension
5	Calf	10-12	2	Standing heel raise	Heel raise
6	Abdomen	35-40	3	Trunk curl	
		10-12	3		Abdominal curl

Note: Week 9 should be followed with a less intense week of training in which weightloads are reduced by 10 pounds and only one set of each exercise is performed.

fifth week provides opportunity for the muscles to recover, adapt, and become stronger. As shown in table 6.7, the strength development exercises remain the same for the second four-week cycle. However, clients' weightloads should increase enough to limit the number of repetitions to those shown in table 6.7. All of the exercises are performed for three sets. During the tenth week, have your clients follow the directions given for week five.

If your clients want more intense split training workouts, refer to the book *Fitness Weight Training* by Baechle and Earle.

Table 6.6

Advanced Muscle Strength Program Weeks 1-4 (First Cycle)					
Order	Muscle group	Reps	Sets	Free-weight	Machine
Upper body exercises: 34 min					
1	*Chest	6-10	3	Bench press	Chest press
2	Chest	8-10	2	Dumbbell fly	Chest crossover
3	*Back	6-10	2	Dumbbell row	Compound row
4	*Shoulder	6-10	3	Standing press	Shoulder press
5	Back	8-10	2	Lat pulldown	Pulldown or pullover
6	Triceps	10	2	Dumbbell triceps extension	Triceps extension
7	Biceps	10	2	Biceps curl	Biceps curl
Lower body exercises: 33 min					
1	*Thigh	6-10	3	Squat	Double leg press
2	*Thigh	6-10	3	Lunge	Single leg press
3	Hamstrings	8-10	2	Leg curl	Leg curl
4	Quadriceps	8-10	2	Leg extension	Leg extension
5	Calf	8-10	2	Standing heel raise	Heel raise
6	Abdomen	30	3	Trunk curl	
		8-10	3		Abdominal curl

*In the exercises marked with an asterisk gradually increase weightloads which will reduce the number of repetitions—from 8-10 down to 6-8—during weeks 3 through 4.

Note: Week 4 should be followed with a less intense week of training in which weightloads are reduced by 10 pounds and only one set of each exercise is performed.

Advanced Muscle Endurance Programs

The first four weeks of the Advanced muscle endurance program in table 6.8 include three sets of 15 reps in seven exercises for three workouts a week. There is one exercise for each of the seven major muscle areas: chest, back, shoulders, biceps, triceps, thighs, and abdomen. During week 5 reduce your client's weightload by 10 pounds and the number of sets to 1, to allow the muscles to recover, adapt, and become stronger. Weeks 6 through 9 include three additional exercises—one each for the chest, back, and calves (see table 6.9). During weeks 6 through 9, progressively increase the number of repetitions to 20. After week 9 repeat the protocol described for week 5.

Table 6.7

Advanced Muscle Strength Program Weeks 6-9 (Second Cycle)

Order	Muscle group	Reps	Sets	Free-weight	Machine
Upper body exercises: 42 min					
1	Chest	5	3	Bench press	Chest press
2	Chest	8-10	3	Dumbbell fly	Chest crossover
3	Back	5	3	Dumbbell row	Compound row
4	Shoulder	5	3	Standing press	Shoulder press
5	Back	8-10	3	Lat pulldown	Pulldown or pullover
6	Triceps	10	3	Dumbbell triceps extension	Triceps extension
7	Biceps	10	3	Biceps curl	Biceps curl
Lower body exercises: 37 min					
1	Thigh	5	3	Squat	Double leg press
2	Thigh	5	3	Lunge	Single leg press
3	Hamstrings	8-10	3	Leg curl	Leg curl
4	Quadriceps	8-10	3	Leg extension	Leg extension
5	Calf	8-10	3	Standing heel raise	Heel raise
6	Abdomen	35-40	3	Trunk curl	
		8-10	3		Abdominal curl

Note: Week 9 should be followed with a less intense week of training in which weightloads are reduced by 10 pounds and only one set of each exercise is performed.

Determining Weightloads for New Exercises

To determine loads for new exercises, follow these guidelines:

1. Show your client how to perform exercises with the lightest weightstack plate (machine exercises), the smallest dumbbell (dumbbell exercises), or with a dowel stick or unloaded bar (barbell exercises), using the teaching strategies described in chapter 3.

2. Identify a weightload you believe will permit 15 repetitions, and ask your client to perform 15 reps.

3. Observe your client's level of effort in performing the number of repetitions completed.

4. Use table 5.5 as a guide for decreasing or increasing weightloads.

Table 6.8

Advanced Muscle Endurance Program
Weeks 1-4 (First Cycle)

Order	Muscle group	Reps	Sets	Free-weight	Machine
				Exercises: 31 min	
1	Chest	15	3	Bench press	Chest press
2	Back	15	3	Dumbbell row	Compound row
3	Shoulder	15	3	Standing press	Shoulder press
4	Biceps	15	3	Biceps curl	Biceps curl
5	Triceps	15	3	Dumbbell triceps extension	Triceps extension
6	Thigh	15	3	Lunge	Double leg press
7	Abdomen	30	3	Trunk curl	
		15	3		Abdominal curl

Table 6.9

Advanced Muscle Endurance Program
Weeks 6-9 (Second Cycle)

Order	Muscle group	Reps	Sets	Free-weight	Machine
				Exercises: 34 min	
1	Chest	15-20	3	Bench press	Chest press
2	Chest	15-20	1	Dumbbell fly	Chest crossover
3	Back	15-20	3	Dumbbell row	Compound row
4	Shoulder	15-20	3	Standing press	Shoulder press
5	Back	15-20	1	Lat pulldown	Pulldown or pullover
6	Triceps	15-20	3	Dumbbell triceps extension	Triceps extension
7	Biceps	15-20	3	Biceps curl	Biceps curl
8	Thigh	15-20	3	Lunge	Double leg press
9	Calf	15-20	3	Standing heel raise	Heel raise
10	Abdomen	40	3	Trunk curl	
		15	3		Abdominal curl

chapter seven

Alternative Exercises and Programs

Although machine and free-weight training offer certain advantages, other forms of resistance equipment can produce excellent results. Weight training equipment intimidates some older adults. For others, budget constraints make membership in a fitness facility or the purchase of strength training equipment impractical. Exercise involving one's own bodyweight and those in which elastic bands are used are effective, convenient, and inexpensive.

Planning Your Prescription

We have grouped both the bodyweight and the elastic band exercises by muscle areas worked, and have arranged them from the less challenging to the more challenging. Instruct your clients to move through the ranges of joint movement shown in the exercises and to perform them in a slow, controlled manner. If some individuals initially cannot perform the entire range of movement, encourage them to move gradually toward the full range, unless doing so will aggravate an existing joint or muscle condition.

Because people vary widely in their strength levels, no specific prescription—for number of reps or thickness of elastic bands—will apply to all clients. Before prescribing an exercise, consider the potential difficulty your client will have in performing the exercise, as well as the resistance he or she must overcome. Table 7.1 provides some helpful guidelines for tailoring the exercise to each client.

Table 7.1

Bodyweight and Elastic Resistance Training Guidelines			
	Fitness Level		
	Low	**Average**	**High**
Exercise or resistance	Permits 5 reps	Permits 10 reps	Permits 15-20 reps
Starting number of sets	1	1	2
Increase sets when reps completed equals	10	15	20-25
Increase sets to	2	2-3	3-4
Rest periods between sets	3 min	2-3 min	1-2 min

Guidelines for Reps, Sets, and Rest Periods

For clients with the lowest strength levels, try to identify which exercises they can perform correctly for at least five repetitions (see table 7.1). For average individuals, identify which exercises can be performed correctly for no more than 10 repetitions. And for those who are most fit, identify exercises that result in fatigue after about 15 or 20 reps. If you are using elastic resistance exercises, select a band or thickness that will accommodate the number of repetitions recommended for the different strength levels in table 7.1. Unless joint or muscle problems preclude certain exercises, try to include at least one exercise for the upper body, one for the lower body, and one for the midsection from those presented later in this chapter. Low strength clients, using a bodyweight program, can use the push-away (wall) for chest and triceps, quarter (depth) knee bend for quadriceps and hamstrings, and the assisted bent-knee trunk curl for abdominal muscles. If clients will be using elastic bands or tubing, they can do the chest press for the chest and triceps, the squat for the quadriceps and hamstrings, and the trunk curl for the abdominals.

Depending on your clients' strength levels, start them out with one or two sets and have them rest one to three minutes between sets. Table 7.1 provides guidelines for progressively increasing the number of sets.

Bodyweight Exercises

Each of the following exercises uses only bodyweight, thereby offering considerable training versatility at no cost. One drawback of bodyweight exercises is that it is difficult to match the appropriate resistance to different strength levels. This chapter includes some variations of traditional exercises that can make bodyweight exercises more practical and productive no matter what your clients' fitness levels. Whichever variations your clients use, see that they perform all exercises through the proper range, in a slow and controlled manner, and that they use the correct body positions shown in the following illustrations.

Push-Up and Push-Up Variations

The basic push-up and its variations are excellent exercises for developing the pectoralis major, anterior deltoid, and triceps muscles. Instruct your clients to keep their backs straight during the basic push-up and its variations. Note that in all push-up exercises (including the push-away), clients should exhale during pushing movements and inhale on return movements.

PUSH-AWAY (WALL)

This is a good exercise for seniors who find standard push-ups too difficult, since it recruits essentially the same muscle groups as the push-up (pectoralis major, anterior deltoid, and triceps). Instruct clients to assume a position in which their feet are about two to three feet from a wall, their hands on the wall are slightly wider than shoulder-width apart, and their elbows are almost fully extended. They should move their chest toward the wall by flexing their elbows, pausing briefly, and then pushing back to the starting position.

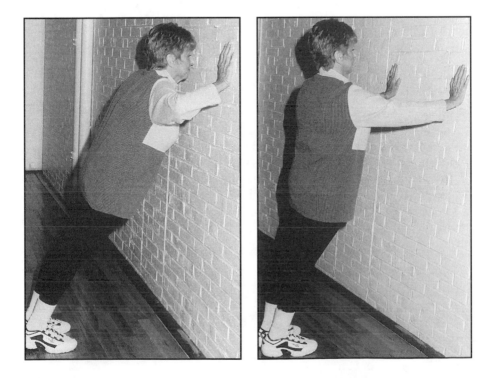

TABLE PUSH-UPS

Instruct clients to stand about four feet from a table, placing their hands slightly more than shoulder-width apart on the table's edge. They should slowly lower their torsos until their chest is near the table. After a momentary pause, they should push back to the starting position. Make sure the table is stable or braced against a wall.

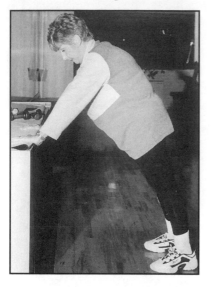
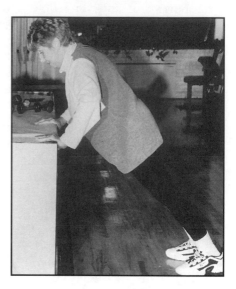

FLOOR PUSH-UPS

While lying on their stomachs, your clients should be instructed to place their hands slightly more than shoulder-width apart on the floor, while maintaining a straight body posture. They should push up to the starting position, pause momentarily, then lower their torsos slowly until their chests near the floor. If the straight body position makes it too difficult for clients to complete at least five repetitions, have them do the push-ups from their knees to reduce the resistance. By instructing them to vary their hand position you can emphasize different muscles: placing the hands farther apart puts more stress on the pectoral muscles, while putting the hands closer together stresses the triceps.

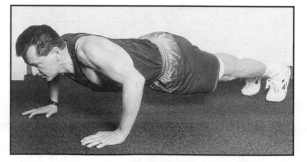

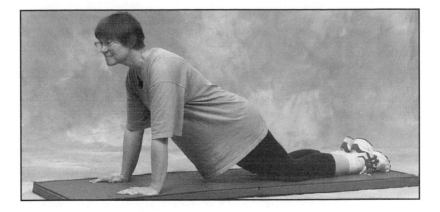

CHAIR PUSH-UPS

When clients are able to complete 15 controlled floor push-ups, you can increase the difficulty by having them put their feet on a stable chair or bench. Their hands slightly wider than shoulder-width apart on the floor, and their bodies straight, they should slowly lower their torsos until their chest nears the floor. After a momentary pause, they should push back up to the starting position.

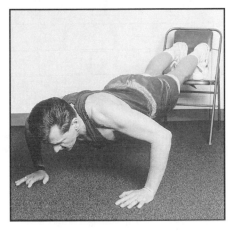

Trunk Curls

Properly performed trunk curls strengthen the abdominal muscles in the front (rectus abdominis) and sides (external and internal obliques) of the midsection. Proper breathing technique during all of the trunk curl exercises involves exhaling during upward movements, and inhaling during downward movements.

ASSISTED BENT-KNEE TRUNK CURL

Instruct clients to assume a supine position on a mat—arms at their sides, and elbows, forearms, and palms in contact with the mat. Knees should be in a flexed position, with heels close to the buttocks. Have your clients initiate the upward curling movement by flexing their trunks and pushing against the mat with their forearms. When their upper backs reach a 30-degree angle, they should pause momentarily before returning to the starting position.

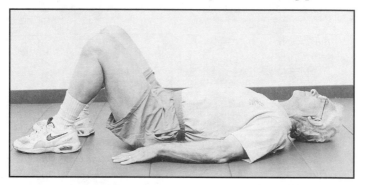

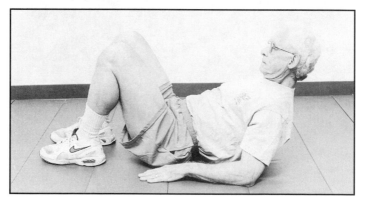

TRUNK CURL WITH BENT KNEES

Have clients assume the position described in the assisted bent-knee trunk curl, but with their hands placed loosely on the sides of their heads to help keep the head and neck in a neutral position. Clients should be instructed to slowly curl their shoulders and upper back off the floor, until the lower back is pressed firmly against the floor. They should pause momentarily before returning to the starting position.

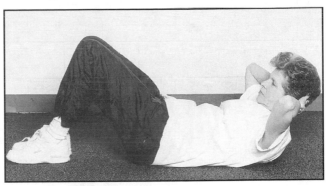

TRUNK CURL WITH KNEE PULL

This exercise is similar to the basic trunk curl, with one additional component: as the trunk curls upward, the exerciser pulls back the left knee in an effort to touch the left elbow. There is a momentary pause before returning to the starting position. The next repetition involves the right knee and right elbow in the same manner. Have your clients alternate the knee-to-elbow action throughout the exercise. The trunk curl with knee pull provides resistance from both the upper and lower body, placing more stress on the abdominal and hip flexor muscles.

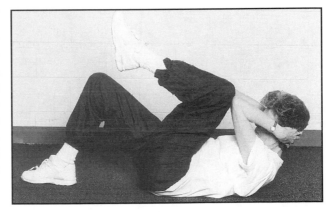

TWISTING TRUNK CURL WITH LEGS ON CHAIR

Clients should be instructed to place their legs on a stable chair or bench as shown below, then curl their shoulders upward off the floor until their lower backs are pressed firmly against the floor—at which time they rotate their trunks to the left or to the right, pausing momentarily before returning to the starting position. They should alternate the direction of the trunk rotations on each repetition. The alternating twists emphasize the muscles on the sides of the midsection (obliques) as well as the rectus abdominis.

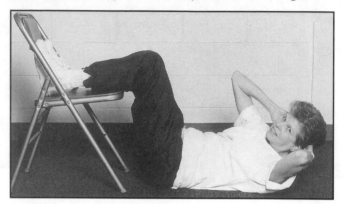

Knee Bends

Knee bends are a good exercise for developing the quadriceps, hamstrings, and gluteal muscle groups. Exhalation in these exercises should occur during upward movement, and inhalation during the downward movements.

QUARTER-KNEE BEND

With feet slightly more than shoulder-width apart and torso erect, clients should be instructed to lower their hips downward and backward to a one-quarter-flexed knee position. They should pause momentarily before returning to the starting position. If maintaining balance is a problem, instruct clients to place one or both hands on a fixed object such as a chair or table. There will be a tendency for the heels to come up as the hips are lowered; however, feet should remain flat on the floor throughout the exercise.

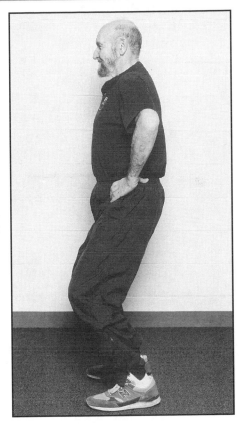

HALF-KNEE BEND

This exercise is identical to the quarter-knee bend, except that the hips are lowered downward and backward to a one-half-flexed knee position. There will be a tendency for the heels to come up as the hips are lowered; however, feet should remain flat on the floor throughout the exercise.

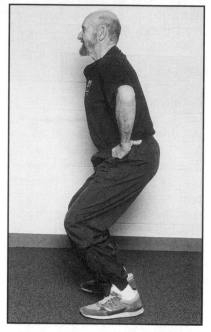

THREE-QUARTER KNEE BEND

This is simply a more demanding version of the half-knee bend because the hips need to be lowered to a three-quarter depth position. This figure illustrates the bottom position of the three-quarter knee bend exercise.

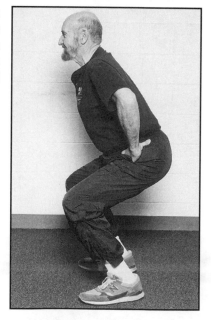

Pull-Ups

Pull-ups develop the latissimus dorsi and biceps muscles. Many people cannot pull up their full bodyweight; but because muscles are stronger in lowering than in lifting movements, almost everyone is able to perform some variation of this exercise. In all pull-up exercises, have your clients use an underhand grip, keep their backs straight, and look straight ahead.

STEP BOX PULL-UP—LOWERING ONLY

Your clients should step onto the box so that their chins are above the bar, grasping it with their palms facing their shoulders, about shoulder-width apart. They should be instructed to slowly lower their bodies until their elbows are fully extended. As soon as their arms are straight, they should return to the starting position by stepping onto the box again. In this exercise, have your clients exhale during the lowering phase and inhale when stepping back onto the box.

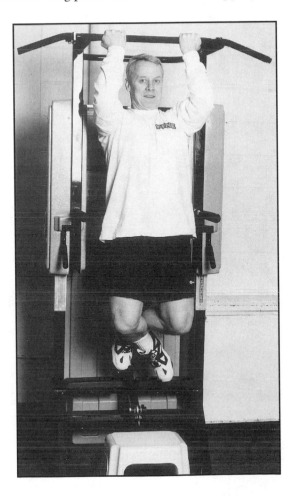

STEP BOX PULL-UP—LEG ASSIST

Have your clients step onto the box and grasp the bar with their palms facing their shoulders, about shoulder-width apart. Then, have them flex their knees so that their elbows are nearly extended. They should use their legs to help lift their bodies during the upward pull-up phase but not during the lowering phase. They should exhale during the upward movement and inhale during the downward movement.

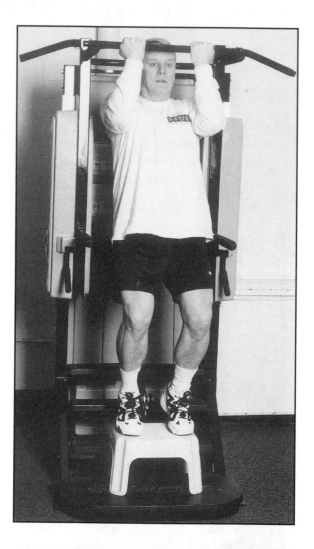

PARTIAL PULL-UP

Have your clients stand on the box and grasp the bar as previously described with their chin above the bar. They slowly lower their bodies until their elbows are one-quarter extended, pausing momentarily before pulling back up to the starting position. Clients should inhale during the lowering movement and exhale during the upward movement. As clients become stronger, you may want to instruct them to lower their bodies until their elbows are extended halfway. The next step is to have them try three-quarter depth repetitions—and, in the final stage, a full-range pull-up.

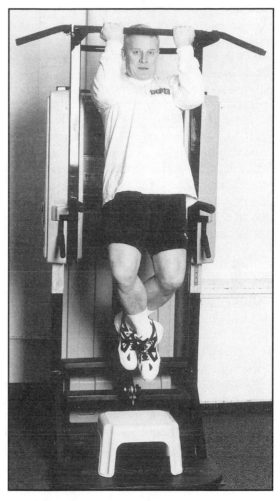

Elastic Resistance Exercises

Another inexpensive and versatile alternative to traditional strength training equipment is resistance bands or tubing. There are some limitations, the first being the difficulty of assigning which lengths and thicknesses of tubing to use. Because there is no standardized system for classifying resistance levels for length and thickness, you must simply use your best judgment in determining what is needed for your client at a given stage. This may not be as difficult as it sounds: through careful observation of your clients, you can gauge pretty well when they are ready to progress to shorter lengths or to greater thicknesses. The main drawback of elastic resistance exercise is that it allows a less objective and observable measure of progress than is available with free weights and weightstack machines. Another limitation is the lack of uniform resistance throughout the movement range: there is less resistance at the start and increased resistance at the end of an exercise when the elastic is stretched the most.

On a positive note, since the bands come in many thicknesses, they offer progressive levels of resistance. You can purchase elastic tubing of various diameters (easily distinguished by different colors) in either pre-cut sections or a roll. We recommend rolls, which you can cut to whatever length you need. You probably should purchase a variety of elastic equipment, from very thin flat bands to thicker round tubing, to accommodate smaller and larger muscle groups, as well as different strength levels. These variations enable you to progressively increase your clients' training intensity in a systematic manner. Elastic equipment offers an excellent training option, especially for training large exercise groups or small exercise areas.

Technique Pointers

Along with teaching your clients when to inhale and exhale, and how to perform repetitions in a controlled manner, you also should instruct them to perform elastic resistance exercises in the proper plane of movement (Purvis 1997). In doing so, they will apply resistance to the muscle group(s) for which the specific exercises are designed; and will also avoid placing inappropriate stress on ligaments and joints.

You may have difficulty determining where to anchor the elastic so that the movement pattern will be in the correct plane. Figures 7.1 through 7.3 illustrate correct and incorrect planes of movement for several exercises. These examples should help you position your client and the anchoring end of the elastic so that the exercise is performed in the proper movement pattern.

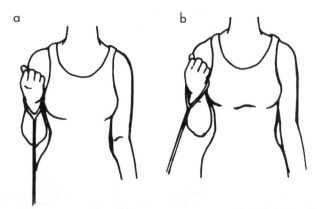

Figure 7.1　(a) Correct, (b) incorrect.

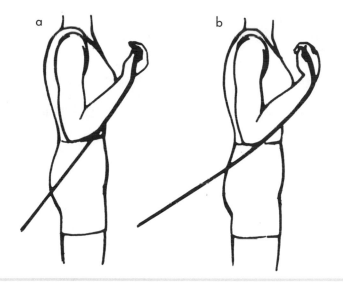

Figure 7.2   (a) Correct, (b) incorrect.

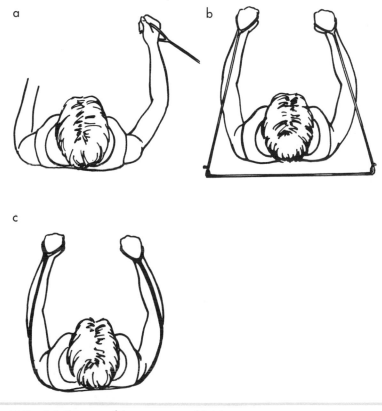

Figure 7.3   (a) Correct, (b) correct, and (c) incorrect.

Safety Precautions

It's also a challenge to figure out *how* to anchor the elastic. Take great care to ensure that it is secure! Try installing hooks in strategic locations in the stud of a wall or in a platform. Only as a last resort should you assign a partner to hold the anchoring end. Due to the skill required of both persons to balance the opposing pulling actions, partner exercises with elastic bands may increase injury risk.

Consider the type and shape of the handle needed for the moving end of the elastic band. Before you purchase or design equipment, analyze the grip requirements of the planned exercises as well as the limitations (e.g., arthritis) of your older adult clients. Purvis (1997) has suggested the use of webbing or mesh that is long enough to fit over the ball of the foot. The same concept is adaptable for almost any situation where your client is unable to grip or otherwise hold onto the end of the elastic band. The four elastic resistance exercises that follow address most of the major muscle groups. When used with the previously described training guidelines, they should provide a good basic workout.

ELASTIC RESISTANCE BAND SQUAT

Like the knee bends previously described, this exercise involves the quadriceps, hamstrings, and gluteal muscles. Instruct your clients to establish a stance slightly wider than shoulder-width, with their feet squarely on the resistance band. They should grasp the handles of the bands so that the bands are taut when your clients are at the three-quarter knee-bend position. From this depth, clients should extend their knees and hips until they are standing up-right. After a momentary pause, they should return slowly to the starting position shown below. Have your clients exhale during the upward movement and inhale during the downward movement.

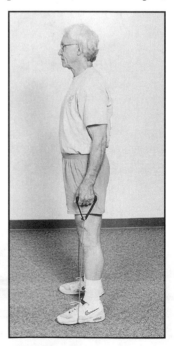

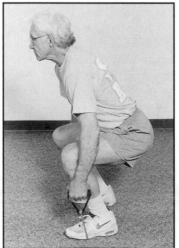

ELASTIC RESISTANCE BAND BENCH PRESS

Like the free-weight bench press, this exercise develops the pectoralis major, anterior deltoid, and triceps muscles. Have clients sit or stand in an upright position with the resistance band or tubing at chest height. The tubing should be attached to a wall hook, although it may be secured adequately to a chair back or a stationary piece of equipment. Instruct clients to hold the handles so that the bands are taut while near the chest before pushing their hands forward. They should push their hands forward until their elbows are almost fully extended, then pause momentarily before returning slowly to the starting position. They should exhale during the pushing phase and inhale during the return movement.

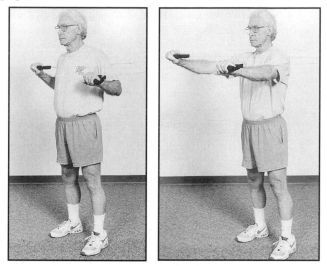

ELASTIC RESISTANCE BAND SEATED ROWS

This exercise primarily works the latissimus dorsi, the rhomboid muscles of the upper back, and the biceps. Have clients sit on the floor with their legs almost straight and torsos erect. Secure the bands to a stationary piece of equipment or to hooks on a wall. They should grasp the band so that it is taut when their arms are extended straight in front. While maintaining an erect torso, clients should pull their hands to their chest, pause momentarily, and then return slowly to the starting position. Instruct clients to exhale during the pulling phase and inhale during the return movement.

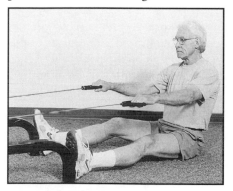 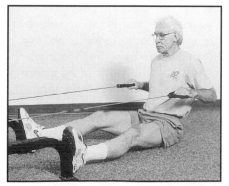

ELASTIC RESISTANCE BICEPS CURL

Like the free-weight biceps curl, this exercise develops primarily the biceps and brachilis muscles. Have clients anchor the band or tubing beneath their feet or onto a floor platform hook and position their feet so that the band or tubing is correctly aligned in the upper position as shown in figure 7.1. The exercise begins from the straight elbow position and ends in the position shown in the figure below. Exhalation should occur during the upward movement, and inhalation during the downward movement.

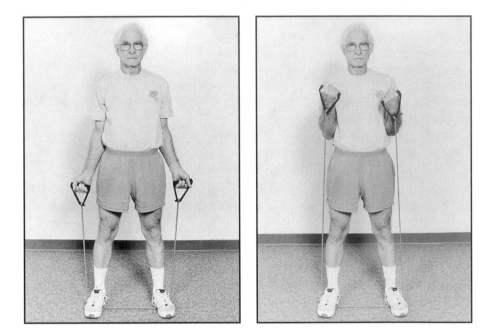

Summary

The exercise procedures described in this chapter should enhance your clients' strength training experiences and reduce the likelihood of injury. These alternatives to free-weight and machine exercises will be especially helpful to instructors who value resistance training for older clients, but have limited access to more expensive equipment. Many exercise options are available to enthusiastic and creative instructors who realize that resistance training can significantly improve the quality of life for senior men and women.

chapter eight

Progress Assessment

For some older adults, informal progress assessments—such as noting weightload increases on their training logs, climbing stairs without difficulty, or observing a more fit appearance in the mirror—may be sufficient. Others may appreciate more formal assessments of their training progress, as well as normative standards against which to evaluate their present level of physical fitness. Four specific areas in which seniors can rate the effectiveness of their exercise program are muscle strength, joint flexibility, body composition, and personal perceptions. Keep in mind that reliable progress assessments depend upon precise testing procedures that are performed in exactly the same manner before and after the training program.

Muscle Strength

Muscle strength is obviously related to the exercise program, and we should expect trained muscles to be stronger than untrained muscles. Strength improvements can be estimated easily by comparing exercise weightloads before and after the training program. Observing personal progress is motivational, and encourages most older adults to continue strength training.

However, many clients also want to know how their strength level compares to other individuals in their age and gender category. For this reason, we have determined normative strength data for men and women between 20 and 80 years of age.

Age and Gender Comparisons

Table 8.1 presents normative information on 245 men and women in their 20s through 70s who were assessed for muscle strength on 13 Nautilus machines

(Westcott 1994). The numbers represent the average exercise weightloads that the subjects could perform for 10 repetitions (10 RM) in good form after two months of regular strength training. Although the weightloads listed in table 8.1 are specific to Nautilus equipment, they should be similar to the weightloads used for the same exercises on other types of weightstack machines.

These data show that the 10-repetition maximum weightloads generally decreased between 5 and 10% every decade, demonstrating a progressive loss of muscle strength throughout the adult years. Also, within each age category, the men's 10-repetition maximum weightloads were approximately 50% higher than the women's.

While men can lift heavier weightloads than women, one large-scale study indicated that both genders are similar in strength on a muscle-for-muscle basis (Westcott 1987).

Table 8.2 shows that male subjects performed 10 leg extensions with 50% more weight than female subjects; but when adjusted for differences in bodyweight (weightload divided by bodyweight), males completed 10 leg extensions with 62% of their bodyweight and females completed 10 leg extensions with 55% of their bodyweight.

When adjusted for differences in lean weight (weightload divided by estimated lean weight), both males and females completed 10 leg extensions with about 75% of their lean weight, suggesting nearly equal quadriceps strength on a muscle-for-muscle basis.

YMCA Leg Extension Test

The individual training programs presented in chapter 5 frequently referred to the client's present level of strength fitness. Our criterion for categorizing a client's strength fitness is the YMCA Leg Extension Test, based on the performance of 907 men and women (Westcott 1987). This easy-to-administer assessment addresses the large and frequently used quadriceps muscles, making it appropriate for older adults. Because it uses the 10-repetition maximum weightload, it is also a safe test, well below the clients' maximum capacity. The YMCA Leg Extension Test also evaluates muscle performance relative to bodyweight, making it a fair strength assessment for men and women of various sizes.

The original strength classifications used in the YMCA Leg Extension Test were derived from scores of men and women in their mid-40s. Modified assessment categories have been developed for men and women in their 50s, 60s, and 70s, based on a study of strength changes over six decades of adult life (Westcott 1994).

The YMCA leg extension test procedures are as follows:

- Select a weightload on a leg extension machine that is about 25% of the client's bodyweight, and encourage the participant to perform 10 repetitions in the following manner:

Table 8.1

	Average Exercise Weightloads on Common Nautilus Machines (N = 245)					

	Age Groups					
Exercises	20-29	30-39	40-49	50-59	60-69	70-79
Leg extension						
Males (lb)	112.5	105.0	97.5	90.0	82.5	75.0
Females (lb)	*67.5*	*65.0*	*62.5*	*60.0*	*57.5*	*55.0*
Leg curl						
Males (lb)	112.5	105.0	97.5	90.0	82.5	75.0
Females (lb)	*67.5*	*65.0*	*62.5*	*60.0*	*57.5*	*55.0*
Leg press						
Males (lb)	240.0	220.0	200.0	180.0	160.0	140.0
Females (lb)	*165.0*	*150.0*	*135.0*	*120.0*	*110.0*	*100.0*
Chest cross						
Males (lb)	100.0	95.0	90.0	85.0	80.0	70.0
Females (lb)	*57.5*	*55.0*	*52.5*	*50.0*	*47.5*	*45.0*
Chest press						
Males (lb)	100.0	102.5	95.0	87.5	80.0	72.5
Females (lb)	*57.5*	*55.0*	*52.5*	*50.0*	*47.5*	*45.0*
Compound row						
Males (lb)	140.0	132.5	125.0	117.5	110.0	102.5
Females (lb)	*85.0*	*82.5*	*80.0*	*77.5*	*75.0*	*70.0*
Shoulder press						
Males (lb)	105.0	97.5	90.0	82.5	72.5	62.5
Females (lb)	*50.0*	*47.5*	*45.0*	*42.5*	*40.0*	*37.5*
Biceps curl						
Males (lb)	90.0	85.0	80.0	75.0	70.0	60.0
Females (lb)	*50.0*	*47.5*	*45.0*	*42.5*	*40.0*	*37.5*
Triceps extension						
Males (lb)	90.0	85.0	80.0	75.0	70.0	60.0
Females (lb)	*50.0*	*47.5*	*45.0*	*42.5*	*40.0*	*37.5*
Low-back						
Males (lb)	110.0	105.0	100.0	95.0	90.0	85.0
Females (lb)	*80.0*	*77.5*	*75.0*	*72.5*	*67.5*	*65.0*
Abdominal curl						
Males (lb)	110.0	105.0	100.0	95.0	90.0	80.0
Females (lb)	*65.0*	*62.5*	*60.0*	*57.5*	*55.0*	*52.5*
Neck flexion						
Males (lb)	70.0	67.5	65.0	62.5	60.0	55.0
Females (lb)	*45.0*	*42.5*	*40.0*	*37.5*	*35.0*	*32.5*
Neck extension						
Males (lb)	80.0	77.5	75.0	72.5	70.0	60.0
Females (lb)	*52.5*	*50.0*	*47.5*	*45.0*	*42.5*	*40.0*

Adapted, by permission, from W. Westcott, 1994, "Strength training for life: Weightloads: Go figure," *Nautilus Magazine* 3(4): 5-7.

Table 8.2

Quadriceps Strength Measured by the 10-Repetition Maximum Weightload on a Nautilus Leg Extension Machine (N = 907)		
	Men	**Women**
Age	43 yr	42 yr
Bodyweight	191 lb	143 lb
10-rep max	119 lb	79 lb
Strength quotient (bodyweight)	62%	55%
Strength quotient (lean bodyweight)	74%	73%

Adapted, by permission, from W. Westcott, 1996, *Building Strength and Stamina* (Champaign, IL: Human Kinetics), 4.

1. Lift the roller pad in 2 seconds to full knee extension.

2. Hold the fully contracted position for 1 second.

3. Lower the roller pad in 4 seconds until the weightstack lightly touches.

• Take a 2-minute rest, select a weightload that is about 35% of the client's bodyweight, and encourage the participant to perform 10 repetitions in the prescribed manner.

• Continue testing with progressively greater resistance until you determine the 10-repetition maximum weightload.

• Divide this weightload by the client's bodyweight to obtain a *strength quotient*, and determine the participant's present strength fitness category (see tables 8.3 and 8.4).

Evaluation by Tracking Progress

If appropriate testing equipment is not available, you can periodically evaluate strength by comparing your client's exercise weightloads over time. As a general rule, weightloads should increase about 45% during the first two months of training, and about 15% during the next two months. Thereafter, a 5% strength gain every two months represents a productive training

Table 8.3

YMCA Leg Extension Test Score Categories for Men

Muscle strength	Ages 50-59 (% bodyweight)	Ages 60-69 (% bodyweight)	Ages 70-79 (% bodyweight)
Low	≤ 44%	≤ 39%	≤ 34%
Below average	45-54%	40-49%	35-44%
Average	55-64%	50-59%	45-54%
Above average	65-74%	60-69%	55-64%
High	≥ 75%	≥ 70%	≥ 65%

Example: A 55-year-old male who weighs 180 pounds and completes 10 leg extensions with 120 pounds has a strength quotient of 66% and *above average* strength in his quadriceps muscles.

Table 8.4

YMCA Leg Extension Test Score Categories for Women

Muscle strength	Ages 50-59 (% bodyweight)	Ages 60-69 (% bodyweight)	Ages 70-79 (% bodyweight)
Low	≤ 34%	≤ 29%	≤ 24%
Below average	35-44%	30-39%	25-34%
Average	45-54%	40-49%	35-44%
Above average	55-64%	50-59%	45-54%
High	≥ 65%	≥ 60%	≥ 55%

Example: A 70-year-old female who weighs 120 pounds and completes 10 leg extensions with 40 pounds has a strength quotient of 33% and *below average* strength in her quadriceps muscles.

program. For example, if a senior male begins with 100 pounds in the leg press, he may be expected to use about 145 pounds (145% of 100) after 8 weeks of training, about 167 pounds (115% of 145) after 16 weeks, and about 175 pounds (105% of 167) after 24 weeks.

Joint Flexibility

Joint flexibility refers to the movement range of a given joint structure, and is related to the muscles' capacity to stretch beyond their resting length. Because poor hip-trunk flexibility may be related to low-back problems, this is the area most frequently evaluated in flexibility tests. Clients with acceptable hip-trunk flexibility should be able to touch their toes without bending their knees; but to reduce the possibility of back strain, have your clients perform this assessment in a sitting position rather than a standing position. This is typically referred to as the sit-and-reach test.

Although specially designed testing devices facilitate assessments of hip-trunk flexibility (figure 8.1), a simple testing procedure requires only a yardstick. After your client warms up, have her sit on the floor with the yardstick between her legs, the 15-inch mark even with her heels. Encourage her to reach forward as far as possible without straining and with the knees straight. Record the farthest reach of three trials, and determine flexibility fitness according to table 8.5.

If your clients can reach the 15-inch mark (by the heels), they are reasonably flexible in the hip-trunk area. If they cannot, an inch per month increase represents an excellent rate of improvement in hip-trunk flexibility.

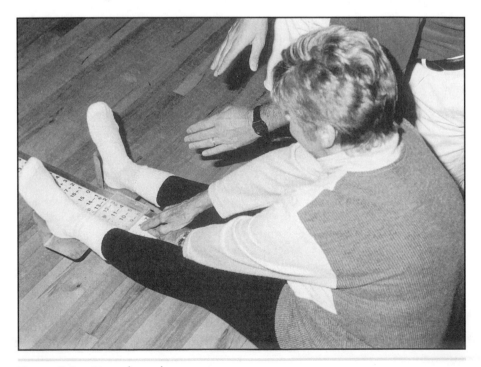

Figure 8.1   Sit-and-reach test.

Table 8.5

Hip-Trunk Flexibility Assessments for Men and Women Over Age 45 Based on Sit-and-Reach Test Scores		
Assessment	**Men (in.)**	**Women (in.)**
Excellent	19-23	21-24
Good	16-18	19-20
Above average	14-15	17-18
Average	12-13	16
Below average	10-11	14-15
Poor	7-9	11-13
Very poor	1-6	4-10

From L. Golding, C. Myers, and W. Sinning, 1989, *Y's Way to Physical Fitness* (Champaign, IL: Human Kinetics), 116, 122. Adapted with permission of the YMCA of the USA, 101 N. Wacker Drive, Chicago, IL 60606.

In one study (Westcott 1995), 48 adult and senior subjects increased their hip-trunk flexibility by 2.5 inches after two months of strength training even though they performed no stretching exercises. The strength exercises produced significant improvements in hip-trunk flexibility, presumably by stretching the hamstrings and low-back muscles during the full-range exercise movements. When the quadriceps muscles move into their fully contracted position during the leg extension exercise, the hamstrings move into their fully stretched position. These findings suggest that properly performed strength training exercises may enhance joint flexibility.

A study by Westcott, Dolan, and Cavicchi (1996) found combined strength training and flexibility exercise effective for significantly increasing movement range in shoulder abduction, hip flexion, and hip extension. Girouard and Hurley (1995) observed significant improvements in shoulder abduction and shoulder flexion following 10 weeks of combined strength training and flexibility exercise. These results indicate that performing both strength and stretching exercises can increase range of movement in selected joint actions.

Body Composition

Body composition is a relative measure of the two basic components of bodyweight—fat weight and lean weight. Fat weight consists solely of fat tissue, whereas lean weight includes muscle, bones, organs, blood, skin, and all other nonfat tissues. The ratio of fat weight to lean weight is usually reported as percent body fat. Ideally, adult males should be about 15% fat weight and

85% lean weight. That is, a 200-pound male with desirable body composition should have about 30 pounds of fat weight and 170 pounds of lean weight.

Because they have greater fat requirements for reproduction purposes, women should have about 25% fat weight and 75% lean weight. In other words, a 120-pound female with a desirable body composition should have about 30 pounds of fat weight and 90 pounds of lean weight.

The most accurate way to assess body composition is underwater weighing. Because the subject must exhale all air and sit totally submerged in a tank of water, however, underwater weighing is too challenging for most senior men and women. The most frequently used method for determining percent body fat is skinfold measurement using calipers—an inexpensive field technique that trained fitness instructors can administer efficiently and effectively (see figure 8.2).

Is it possible to evaluate progress in overweight adults without the use of body composition assessment equipment? Yes—but bodyweight measurements alone may not be very helpful. For example, a senior who adds 4 pounds of muscle and loses 4 pounds of fat will weigh exactly the same in spite of an 8-pound improvement in body composition. One way to monitor improvements in body composition is to take periodic midsection measurements. Have the subject stand tall, and place a measuring tape around the waist just above

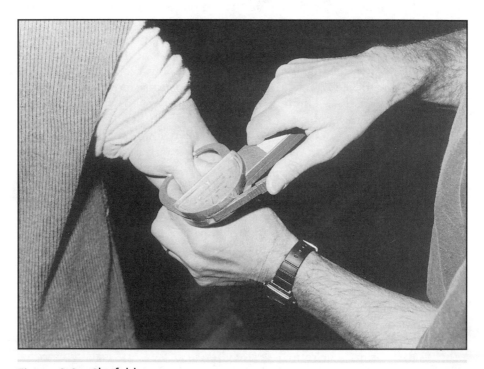

Figure 8.2   Skinfold measurement test.

the belt. A one-half inch reduction in waist girth every month indicates an excellent rate of body composition improvement and a successful strength training program.

Personal Perceptions

It is relatively simple to assess physical improvements in which we can make fairly precise before-and-after measurements—muscle strength, joint flexibility, and body composition. But in some respects, psychological outcomes may be even more important to seniors than physical progress. Are your clients' personal perceptions more positive as a result of their strength training programs? Ideally, older adults should not only be stronger, but should feel better, have more self-confidence, and function more independently after the exercise program.

Although personal perceptions are not easy to quantify, a brief questionnaire may serve this purpose satisfactorily. Consider using the following "Lifestyle Questionnaire" (Westcott 1995) in which participants rate themselves on several fitness-related parameters, recording their physical and personal perceptions on a 5-point scale: low, below average, average, above average, or high. The questionnaire is administered before and after the training program to identify the participants' perceptual changes.

After an eight-week program of strength and endurance exercise, participants in the Westcott (1995) study reported perceived improvements in muscle strength, cardiovascular endurance, joint flexibility, overall physical fitness, coordination, energy level, activity level, and self-confidence. These positive perceptions reinforced the beneficial effects of their exercise efforts, and encouraged over 90% of the participants to continue their fitness program. If you choose to use the Lifestyle Questionnaire with your own clients, you may want to copy it at 145% to obtain an 8.5" × 11" version. For further information on personal perceptions and exercise adherence, we recommend Rod Dishman's excellent text *Exercise Adherence* (Human Kinetics).

Summary of Rating Processes

Some seniors are content to evaluate their strength training program by noting weightload increases in their training log. Others prefer formal assessments of their progress, and some want specific feedback that enables them to compare their fitness level to that of their peers.

- The YMCA Leg Extension Test effectively and safely measures *lower body muscle strength*, providing research-based ratings of muscle strength for men and women in their 50s, 60s, and 70s. The test evaluates the large quadriceps muscles, relative to the subject's bodyweight, using the 10-repetition maximum weightload.

Lifestyle Questionnaire

Age _____   Gender _____   Date _____

Please indicate the most accurate response to each of the following questions. Thank you.

	High	Above average	Average	Below average	Low
1. My overall level of physical fitness is . . .	❑	❑	❑	❑	❑
2. My level of muscular strength is . . .	❑	❑	❑	❑	❑
3. My level of cardiovascular endurance is . . .	❑	❑	❑	❑	❑
4. My level of joint flexibility is . . .	❑	❑	❑	❑	❑
5. My general energy level is . . .	❑	❑	❑	❑	❑
6. My daily activity level is . . .	❑	❑	❑	❑	❑
7. My desire to do physical activities is . . .	❑	❑	❑	❑	❑
8. My ability to walk a mile is . . .	❑	❑	❑	❑	❑
9. My ability to lift and carry large objects (groceries, suitcases, vacuum cleaners, etc.) is . . .	❑	❑	❑	❑	❑
10. My level of self-confidence is . . .	❑	❑	❑	❑	❑
11. My level of personal independence is . . .	❑	❑	❑	❑	❑
12. My level of coordination is . . .	❑	❑	❑	❑	❑

Source: South Shore YMCA Fitness Research Department.

• You can assess *joint flexibility* with the sit-and-reach test. This evaluation targets the hip and trunk muscles, which are closely related to low-back health. Research indicates that properly performed strength exercise improves hip and trunk flexibility.

• Body composition refers to the ratio of fat weight to lean weight, and is usually reported as percent body fat. The most common and practical method for assessing *percent body fat* is skinfold measurements using calipers. Regular strength training improves body composition by increasing lean weight and decreasing fat weight.

• We suggest administering self-rating questionnaires before and after exercise programs in order to assess *personal perceptions* of fitness-related parameters. Preliminary results indicate that strength training improves older adults' perceptions of their fitness and performance levels, as well as their self-confidence.

chapter nine

Working With Special Populations

The aging process is associated with a variety of diseases and disabilities that make it difficult for some older adults to follow standard strength training programs. This chapter discusses common medical conditions of senior men and women, and suggests sensible modifications that should enable them to strength train safely. We begin with obesity, a problem for one out of three Americans, and a predisposing factor for many older adult disorders. The following sections address diabetes, cardiovascular disease, osteoporosis, low-back pain, arthritis, depression, visual and auditory impairments, as well as general frailty.

Obesity

Approximately 75% of American adults are overweight (Hargrove 1996). People must be more than 20% heavier than recommended bodyweight to be considered obese—yet bodyweight assessments may seriously *under*estimate a person's actual fat content. It is easy to understand why so many senior men and women are debilitated by obesity—they simply have too much fat and too little muscle, which is like driving a tanker truck with a motor scooter engine.

Because nonexercising adults lose over 5 pounds of muscle and add about 15 pounds of fat each decade, their increase in body fat may be 50% greater than their increase in bodyweight (Evans and Rosenberg 1992).

Obese individuals have difficulty moving their bodies, including getting up, getting down, and engaging in all types of ambulatory activities. This is why obese adults typically prefer stationary cycles that support their weight, instead of treadmills and stairclimbing machines that do not. The same reasoning applies to modes of strength training. Whenever possible, obese individuals should begin training with strength exercises that support their bodyweight.

Obesity: Training Protocols

Well-designed strength training machines support the exerciser's weight, as do many free-weight exercises. For example, machine leg presses are preferable to barbell squats for obese exercisers; and seated dumbbell presses and curls are more appropriate free-weight exercises than the standing versions of those exercises.

Obese individuals typically avoid calisthenic exercises such as sit-ups, push-ups, and pull-ups, because their excess bodyweight severely limits the number of repetitions they can perform. Training with machines or free weights avoids this problem, as resistance can be easily adjusted to each exerciser's strength level. For example, the abdominal machine can effectively work the sit-up muscles, free-weight bench presses can fully exercise the push-up muscles, and the weight-assisted chin-dip machine is nearly identical in its effects to actual pull-ups and bar dips.

While cardiovascular exercise is an important component of overall fitness programs, many obese adults find it hard to complete endurance activities. Yet most overweight seniors can successfully perform strength exercises with little difficulty (other than possibly requiring a little assistance getting on and off certain machines or benches), thus providing positive reinforcement to their training efforts.

Given that many older adults suffer from obesity, and even those who are not excessively overweight typically have too much fat and too little muscle, strength training is a desirable activity for seniors because it reduces fat and replaces muscle. You can adjust training resistances for essentially all strength levels, and your clients can perform the exercises on supportive machines or benches.

You should also discuss food intake with overweight clients. Chapter 10 presents important information on proper nutrition, including food selection and substitution for heart-healthy eating that you should know in order to help obese older adults better understand how to attain a more desirable bodyweight.

Diabetes

Diabetes mellitus, commonly called diabetes, is a metabolic dysfunction that prevents glucose, the body's primary fuel source, from being efficiently transported and utilized. In Type I diabetes, the pancreas does not produce enough insulin, the hormone responsible for getting glucose into the body cells. In Type II diabetes, the pancreas manufactures sufficient insulin but the body cells become resistant to its effects. According to Dr. David Nathan, director of the diabetes center at Massachusetts General Hospital, diabetes is difficult to treat once it develops, and is the leading cause of blindness, kidney failure, and limb amputations, as well as a predisposing factor in heart disease and stroke (Foreman 1997).

Genetic factors appear to be involved in some cases of Type II diabetes; but age, impaired glucose tolerance, and obesity are major predisposing factors. Dr. Nathan's research reveals that this disease is about six times more common in adults over age 45 than in those aged 30 through 44. Individuals with impaired glucose tolerance have about a 50% greater chance of developing diabetes than do others. Finally, the risk essentially doubles for people with impaired glucose tolerance who are also obese.

Because all older adults have one risk factor for developing diabetes (age), many have a second (obesity), and some have a third (impaired glucose tolerance), it is prudent to take preventive measures with all of your clients. While most diabetes publications rightly recommend endurance exercise, such as walking (Weil 1993), there is growing interest in adding strength training to the overall fitness program.

> *"Recently, the benefits of incorporating strength training into an overall activity regimen (that includes aerobic activity) for the prevention and treatment of type II diabetes are being recognized."* (President's Council on Physical Fitness and Sports Research Digest, *June 1997*)

Eriksson et al. (1997) showed that strength training significantly improved glycemic control in seniors with Type II diabetes. In addition to increasing glucose utilization, strength training may be the best means for improving body composition and reversing many aspects of the aging process (see chapter 1). But how much strength exercise is necessary, and at what level of intensity should it be performed?

Diabetes: Training Protocols

Based on information currently available, we believe that a basic program of strength exercise is appropriate for people with diabetes, contingent upon physician approval. There is no evidence that strength training has any adverse effects on diabetes, or that high intensity exercise is harmful. In fact, studies with diabetics indicate that higher intensity exercises may be better than lower intensity activities for producing desirable metabolic changes (*President's Council on Physical Fitness and Sports Research Digest* 1997).

We recommend that older adults with diabetes follow the introductory strength training program presented in chapter 5. As they attain greater strength and muscle development, they may progress to one of the more advanced training protocols described in chapter 6.

The major caution when training insulin dependent diabetics is to counter the possibility of acute low blood sugar (hypoglycemia) resulting from the combined effects of insulin supplementation and exercise. Always maintain a supply of canned fruit juice in your activity area. Any client who shows signs of an adverse insulin reaction (such as disorientation or lack of coordination) should immediately sit down and drink six to eight ounces of fruit juice, or consume some other significant source of sugar (Rimmer 1997). Diabetics, like all other exercisers, should drink plenty of fluids before, during, and after each strength training workout.

Cardiovascular Disease

Cardiovascular disease is the leading cause of death in the United States, and is prevalent among many older adults at varying levels of physical impairment. Cardiac patients with unstable conditions, as well as those who have not received physician release from a monitored rehabilitation program, should exercise only under direct medical supervision (Clark 1997). Cardiac patients who are cleared for medically supervised strength training should exercise in accordance with the information obtained from their symptom-limited stress test. Traditionally, postcoronary patients have been advised to begin strength training with about 40% of their maximum resistance (40% of 1 RM) in each exercise (Drought 1995; Kelemen et al. 1986; Vander et al. 1986). Twelve to fifteen repetitions are generally recommended, so long as the patient's effort level does not exceed a *somewhat hard* rating on the Borg (1998) scale of perceived exertion.

After a successful response to the initial strength training program, physicians may prescribe progressively heavier weightloads and eliminate the requirement for medically monitored exercise sessions. For example, the American Association of Cardiovascular and Pulmonary Rehabilitation *Guidelines for Cardiac Rehabilitation Programs* (1995) recommend training weightloads that can be *comfortably* performed for one set of 10-15 repetitions. This typically corresponds to about 60% of the patient's maximum resistance (60% of 1 RM).

Percent 1 RM and Heart Rate

Although cardiac patients should not perform higher percentages of maximum resistance without their physician's permission, workloads up to 80% of maximum may be safe for many postcoronary participants (Faigenbaum et al. 1990; Ghilarducci, Holly, and Amsterdam 1989). In one study, healthy middle-aged adults completed about 13 repetitions to muscle fatigue with 70% of their maximum weightload (Westcott and O'Grady 1998). On average, this raised their heart rate about 50 beats above resting, to approximately 69% of maximum heart rate. Each repetition at 70% of 1 RM elevated their heart rate about four beats. These same adults completed about seven repetitions to muscle fatigue with 85% of their maximum weightload. As with 70% of the 1 RM, their heart rate increased about 50 beats above resting to approximately 69% of maximum heart rate. However, with the heavier resistance each repetition raised their heart rate about seven beats.

Although both the lighter (70% 1 RM) and heavier (85% 1 RM) weightloads produced about a 50-beat increase in heart rate, the lighter resistance did so in smaller increments. Because lighter weightloads offer more control over cardiovascular responses on a repetition by repetition basis, it makes sense for postcoronary exercisers to begin with low resistance (40 to 60% 1 RM) and progress gradually to higher levels. It is probably unnecessary for cardiac patients to train with more than 70% of maximum weightload, as this resistance level has been shown to produce significant muscle strength development in healthy adults of all ages (Westcott and Guy 1996).

One Approach to Strengthening Muscles of Stroke Clients: When we were asked to rehabilitate former National Football League rushing champion Jim Nance, we didn't know how to strengthen the limbs affected by his stroke. How do you apply resistance to a hand that can't grip and an arm that can't move? We first learned that a velcro glove enabled Jim to hold the handle of the biceps curl machine. We then discovered that, although Jim could not lift any amount of resistance (concentric muscle action), he could lower a little resistance (eccentric muscle action) after we placed his arm in the fully contracted, flexed-elbow position. By progressively training with the eccentric muscle action, Jim gradually increased his biceps strength until he was eventually able to lower and lift relatively heavy weightloads. You may find this training procedure effective for clients with similar disabilities. Just be patient with their progress, especially in the early stages of the exercise program. We suggest following the standard strength training protocol, except that you perform the lifting movements and your client performs the lowering movements.

Training Considerations—AACVPR and ASFA Guidelines

In addition to training with appropriate weightloads, older adult clients with cardiovascular disease should observe the following exercise guidelines taken from the American Association of Cardiovascular and Pulmonary Rehabilitation (1995) and the American Senior Fitness Association (Clark 1997).

- Warm up and cool down thoroughly before and after each strength training session.
- Monitor heart rate and perceived exertion throughout each strength workout.
- Breathe continuously during every repetition, never holding the breath.

- Move the resistance continuously during every repetition, never holding the weight in a static position.
- Hold the resistance with a relaxed grip, never with excessive pressure.
- Use controlled movement speed and full movement range, lifting the resistance in two seconds and lowering it in four seconds.
- Increase the weightloads gradually, by 2.5 pounds when 15 repetitions can be comfortably completed with proper form.
- Keep overhead exercises to a minimum, especially during the early stages of strength training.
- Perform exercises for all of the major muscle groups, following a general sequence from larger to smaller muscles.
- Do two or three strength workouts per week, with at least 48 hours between training sessions.
- Discontinue exercising at the first sign of cardiovascular contraindication, including dizziness, abnormal heart rhythm, unusual shortness of breath, or chest discomfort.

Most cardiac patients can safely perform strength training exercises if they adhere to the training guidelines presented in this chapter and to their physician's recommendations. It is important that they do so to regain strength for performing daily activities without undue exertion or stress on their hearts.

Cardiovascular Disease: Training Protocols

The introductory strength training program presented in chapter 5 meets the exercise guidelines and should work well for most people with cardiovascular disease. Just keep in mind that the suggested starting weightloads in chapter 5 represent about 75% of maximum weightload and should be reduced accordingly for cardiac patients. Lowering the weightloads listed by 10 to 20 pounds should provide appropriate starting levels for most postcoronary participants.

Osteoporosis

There are few physical disorders that have a higher correlation with muscle weakness than osteoporosis. Fortunately, the opposite relationship is true: strong muscles are associated with strong bones (Hughes et al. 1995); and strength training can increase bone mineral density in men and women over 50 years of age (Menkes et al. 1993; Nelson et al. 1994). Dr. Robert A. Gurtler, fellow of both the American Academy of Orthopaedic Surgeons and the American Orthopedic Society of Sports Medicine, says, "Both having the right genetics and practicing good eating habits are essential for the prevention of osteoporosis. But an equally important factor is whether you perform weight-bearing exercise on a regular basis" (personal communication, May 1998).

In a Tufts University study (Nelson et al. 1994), 20 postmenopausal women increased their bone mineral density by 1% after one year of strength training, whereas bone mineral density decreased by 2% during the same period for 19 inactive women. All strength exercises were performed at a high level of intensity, namely, 80% of the 1 RM.

Other Tufts University studies with older men (Frontera et al. 1988) and with women in their nineties (Fiatarone et al. 1990) have also demonstrated excellent results training with 80% of maximum resistance. However, similar increases in muscle mass have been demonstrated with weightloads of 70 to 80% of 1 RM (Westcott and Guy 1996), indicating that a range of resistance may be effective for musculoskeletal development.

Osteoporosis: Training Protocols

We recommend that men and women with osteoporosis train with 70 to 80% of their maximum resistance. This corresponds to a weightload that can be lifted for 8-12 repetitions to muscle fatigue. However, as in the Nelson et al. study (1994), we suggest starting with 50 to 60% of maximum resistance before progressing to heavier workloads.

You can generally apply basic strength training guidelines to people with osteoporosis. Have individuals with very weak bones use very light resistance, preferably training on machines or benches that provide hip and back support; and have them avoid spinal flexion exercises, which may cause fractures (Clark 1997).

Low Back Pain

Affecting four out of five adults, low back pain is a major malady among older men and women. Researchers at the University of Florida have demonstrated that isolated trunk extension exercise increases strength and decreases pain in the low-back area (Risch et al. 1993). Resistance exercises that provide full-range trunk extension and minimize hip extension are most productive for strengthening the low-back muscles (Jones et al. 1988).

> *While it is not advisable to exercise during periods of discomfort, strength training appears to be an effective means for rehabilitating, as well as preventing, low back problems.*

We recommend that people with low back pain first consult their physicians regarding participation in a strength training program. If approved, such people should start with the basic exercises presented in chapter 4, but at reduced resistance. Eliminate from their training protocols any exercise that causes low-back discomfort.

Low Back Pain: Training Protocols

The recommended machine low-back exercise in chapter 4 (see page 64) targets the trunk extensor muscles and de-emphasizes the hip extensor muscles, thereby enhancing low-back strength development. Although the recommended free-weight exercise in chapter 4 is not quite as effective for strengthening the low-back muscles, the trunk extension is an acceptable substitute. This simple exercise uses the low-back muscles to raise the torso from a hip-supported prone position on the floor. By using their arms for assistance, even people with weak low-back muscles should be able to perform this movement productively. Please see page 66 for a detailed description of the trunk extension.

Low-back patients at the University of Florida have experienced excellent results by performing one set of 8 to 12 machine trunk extensions, two or three days per week (Risch et al. 1993), and we recommend a similar training protocol. Unfortunately, not everyone with low-back discomfort is helped by strength training, so it is important to monitor each person's response to every workout. Ideally, the strength training program will be effective, the low-back discomfort will diminish, and the participants will progress to more advanced exercise protocols.

Arthritis

According to the Arthritis Foundation (1997), arthritis refers to more than 100 diseases that cause pain, swelling, and movement restrictions in joints and connective tissue throughout the body. The three most prevalent forms of arthritis are osteoarthritis, rheumatoid arthritis, and fibromyalgia. Because one in seven Americans has arthritis, it is frequently a limiting factor for older adult strength training.

Physicians traditionally have cautioned arthritis sufferers to avoid strenuous exercise in general and strength training in particular. That practice is changing, however, thanks to recent research. For example, a Tufts University study (*Tufts University Diet and Nutrition Letter* 1994) found that 12 weeks of strength training eased the pain of osteoarthritis and rheumatoid arthritis. Program participants performed all of the strength exercises at 80% of their maximum resistance, a relatively high training intensity.

The July-August 1997 issue of *Arthritis Today* featured a detailed article by Dorothy Foltz-Gray on the benefits and procedures for strength training with arthritic individuals. She made the following recommendations:

- Consult with a medical specialist before beginning a strength training program.
- Warm up before strength training to avoid exercising cold joints.
- Cut back on strength training during periods of acute inflammation.

- Evaluate pain the day after strength exercise, and make appropriate adjustments to avoid overtraining.
- Avoid overemphasis on specific areas, and work toward comprehensive muscle conditioning.
- Protect stressed joints by using machines or wrist straps, for example, rather than gripping barbells with arthritic fingers.
- Organize the training program, when appropriate, to avoid unnecessary movements between exercise stations or to avoid sitting and standing exercises.
- Use proper posture to enhance joint function during strength exercise.

According to Janie Clark (1997), President of the American Senior Fitness Association, most strength exercises can be modified to decrease arthritic discomfort and increase ease of execution.

If an exercise causes joint pain that persists for more than one hour it should be replaced. Clark also advises that brief exercise sessions are better tolerated than long workouts. For example, instead of combining strength exercise and aerobic activity into a one-hour workout on Mondays, Wednesdays, and Fridays, people with arthritis may respond more favorably to 30 minutes of strength exercise on Mondays, Wednesdays, and Fridays and 30 minutes of aerobic activity on Tuesdays, Thursdays, and Saturdays.

Arthritis: Training Protocols

We suggest that the basic strength training program presented in chapter 5 is a good starting point for many individuals with arthritis. They may prefer machine training over free weights, since machines provide supportive structures and include fewer exercises that require firm gripping.

Depression

Strength training can improve self-concept in children (Faigenbaum et al. 1997) and increase self-confidence in adults (Westcott 1995). In a recent study conducted at Harvard Medical School (Singh, Clements, and Fiatarone 1997), strength training resulted in significantly reduced depression levels in people over 60 years of age. Of 16 clinically depressed subjects, 14 no longer met the criteria for depression following 10 weeks of strength training.

An important outcome of this study was the finding that participants who trained at higher levels of intensity (more than 80% of maximum resistance) made significantly more improvement in their depression scores than those who trained at lower levels (less than 80% of 1 RM).

Depression: Training Protocols

It appears that depressed older adults may safely and successfully participate in supervised strength training programs. We recommend starting with the standard exercise program presented in chapter 5 and progressing to more advanced programs when appropriate. However, since higher training intensities may be more effective for reducing depression (Singh, Clements, and Fiatarone 1997), we suggest raising the resistance when 10 repetitions (rather than 12) are completed in two consecutive workouts. If the response to this training protocol is positive, consider increasing the weightload when eight repetitions are completed in two successive sessions. Because most people can perform eight repetitions with about 80% of their maximum resistance, this should ensure a relatively high training effort.

Visual and Auditory Impairments

Although most older adults with visual and auditory limitations can learn to strength train independently, you can follow certain procedures and precautions to enhance their experiences.

A good starting point is to make sure the exercise facility has ample lighting and good acoustics. Remove barriers that could cause a fall or collision: clear walkways and workout areas of weights and obstacles, and see that doors are not left half open. Place apparatus with cables and hanging bars, such as lat pulldown machines, in an unobtrusive location, separated from other equipment in general workout areas.

You should provide particularly clear exercise explanations for visually impaired participants, and present precise exercise demonstrations for those with hearing difficulties. Because many people with impaired hearing read lips, be sure to face your clients as much as possible, and speak a little more slowly than usual if you tend to talk quickly (Clark 1997).

Avoid exercises that produce unnecessary pressure in the eyes, as well as actions that elevate blood pressure excessively—holding the breath, holding the resistance in a static position, or straining to complete a final repetition. As both visually and auditorily impaired individuals may have difficulty with balance and postural alignments, we suggest starting with machines or free-weight exercises that can be performed from supported positions. For example, incline bench dumbbell presses are preferable to standing dumbbell presses.

Visual and Auditory Impairments: Training Protocols

You should develop and follow a consistent pattern of exercise sequencing, moving from station to station in a routine manner. Introduce additional exercises one at a time, and take care to establish new movement procedures and pathways around the training facility.

We recommend that older adults with visual or auditory impairment attempt the standard training program presented in chapter 5, assuming the exercise stations are arranged appropriately and are easy to access. Although you may need to make minor exercise adjustments along the way, the training progressions should not be problematic, and improvements in strength should be no different from those of other older adults.

General Frailty

For some older adults, especially in higher age categories, the major physical problem is general frailty—years of inactivity have resulted in severe muscle atrophy and strength loss. Fortunately, Tufts University research with nonagenarians demonstrates that even the oldest and weakest adults respond positively to properly designed strength exercise (Fiatarone et al. 1990).

The Tufts University strength training studies with older adults (Campbell et al. 1994; Fiatarone et al. 1990; Frontera et al. 1988; Nelson et al. 1994) are noted for using heavy weightloads and high-intensity training procedures. The researchers have reported significant musculoskeletal improvements in the participants with no exercise-related injuries.

The Tufts strength training studies have used 80% of maximum resistance and a three-set training protocol. The South Shore YMCA studies (Westcott, Dolan, and Cavicchi 1996; Westcott and Guy 1996) have used a slightly lower exercise resistance (between 70 to 80% of maximum) and a single-set training protocol. Both approaches have produced similar gains in older adults' lean weight. Subjects in the Campbell et al. study (1994) added about 3 pounds of lean weight in three months, while those in the Westcott and Guy study (1996) added about 2.5 pounds of lean weight in two months.

General Frailty: Training Protocols

We recommend that frail older adults begin strength training using single sets, lower weightloads, and fewer exercises, such as the four exercise program presented in the beginning of chapter 5. As they become stronger, and are able to train harder and longer, they may progress to additional sets, heavier weightloads, and more exercises. If necessary, you can modify standard machine and free-weight exercises, or replace them with other resistance devices such as elastic bands.

Summary

Older adults comprise several special populations based on physiological factors and disease states. These include obesity, diabetes, cardiovascular disease, osteoporosis, low-back pain, arthritis, depression, visual and auditory impairments, and general frailty.

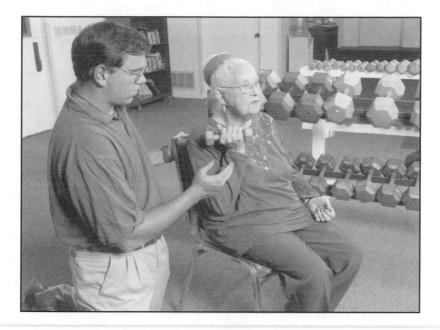

Figure 9.1 Even frail clients can benefit from sensible strength training.

Research indicates that most older adults in these special categories can safely and successfully perform properly designed strength exercises. Perhaps more important, sensible strength training can actually improve many of these debilitating conditions (obesity, osteoporosis, low-back pain, arthritis, depression, and general frailty) and be beneficial in others (diabetes and cardiovascular disease).

Your strength training program should incorporate certain precautions for particular problems, as detailed in the present chapter. Yet the basic training principles of chapter 3 and the standard exercise programs of chapter 5 are generally applicable, even though the workout intensities may be lower and the rates of progression slower.

chapter ten

Nutrition for Senior Weight Trainers

Dietary habits significantly affect your client's bodyweight, body composition, and physical health. Because most Americans consume too many calories for their level of activity, about three out of four adults are overweight (Hargrove 1996)—predisposing them to various diseases and degenerative problems. Your clients should be aware that excessive body fat increases the risk of heart disease, joint problems, diabetes, low-back pain, and many types of cancer.

> *Understanding the problem is only the first step in making lifestyle changes that can lead to a more desirable bodyweight. The physical improvements that result from strength training will motivate some seniors to modify their eating habits in order to further enhance their body composition and personal appearance. Others may need specific nutrition programs that present daily menus and dietary information. Two of the best resources in this area are Nancy Clark's* Sports Nutrition Guidebook *(Human Kinetics Publishers) and Dr. Ellington Darden's* Living Longer Stronger *(Perigee Publishers).*

In addition to knowing how to count calories and determine the fat content of various foods, older adults should be aware that eating too little protein or calcium can lead to a weak musculoskeletal system and even osteoporosis. Insufficient iron in the diet may cause anemia, and excessive sodium intake may contribute to hypertension.

Eating foods high in fiber, low in fat, and rich in vitamins and minerals is essential for optimum health as well as for disease prevention. For example, potassium, which is abundant in bananas and cantaloupe, is involved in every muscle contraction. Vitamins A and C, found in many fruits and vegetables, are important antioxidants (nutritional bodyguards) that protect the body cells from potentially harmful chemical reactions.

While nutritional supplements can supply vitamins and minerals, dieticians recommend that such supplements are not a substitute for well balanced diets that include a variety of vegetables, fruits, and whole grains, as well as lean meats and low-fat dairy products. Human nutrient requirements are too complex (and too little understood) to be adequately supported by pills, and only a varied and well-rounded diet can provide the proper foundation for optimum nutrition. Your clients should be familiar with the food categories and daily servings recommended by the United States Department of Agriculture in the Food Guide Pyramid. They should also understand that a well-balanced diet is not the same as a low-calorie diet designed for losing weight. Be sure your client's physician or a registered dietician approves any reduced-calorie diet .

The Basic Nutrients

The Food Guide Pyramid (figure 10.1) is high in carbohydrates, moderate in proteins, and low in fats. The carbohydrate choices are divided into grains, vegetables, and fruits. The suggested protein sources are low-fat milk products and lean meats, and the recommended fat-rich foods are vegetable oils (used sparingly). Let's consider each of the food categories more carefully.

Grains

Grains include all kinds of foods made from wheat, oats, corn, rice, and the like. Examples of grain foods are cereals, breads, pasta, pancakes, rice cakes, tortillas, bagels, muffins, cornbread, rice pudding, and chocolate cake. Obviously, some grain-based foods such as cakes, cookies, and pastries contain a lot of fat, and should be eaten in moderation.

All grains are high in carbohydrates; some grains, or parts of grains, such as wheat germ, are also good sources of proteins. Whole grains are typically rich in B vitamins and fiber. Grains are plentiful and inexpensive and should be part of every meal—the Food Guide Pyramid recommends 6 to 11 servings of grains every day. A serving is equivalent to a slice of bread or a half cup of pasta, so achieving the 6 to 11 servings should not be too difficult for most clients. Refer to page 197 for sample exchange units for popular food choices within the grains category.

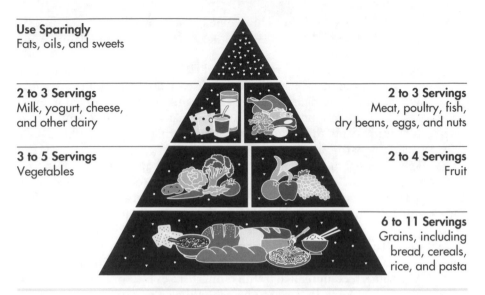

Use Sparingly
Fats, oils, and sweets

2 to 3 Servings
Milk, yogurt, cheese,
and other dairy

2 to 3 Servings
Meat, poultry, fish,
dry beans, eggs, and nuts

3 to 5 Servings
Vegetables

2 to 4 Servings
Fruit

6 to 11 Servings
Grains, including
bread, cereals,
rice, and pasta

Figure 10.1   United States Department of Agriculture Food Guide Pyramid.
United States Departments of Agriculture and Health and Human Services

Vegetables

Like grains, vegetables are excellent sources of carbohydrates, vitamins, and fiber. Vegetables come in all sizes, shapes, colors, and nutritional characteristics, and are relatively low in calories.

• Orange vegetables (e.g., carrots, sweet potatoes, and winter squash) are typically good sources of vitamin A and beta-carotene.

• Green vegetables are characteristically high in vitamins B2 and folic acid. Some of the many green vegetables are peas, beans, broccoli, asparagus, spinach, and lettuce.

• Red vegetables generally provide ample amounts of vitamin C. The best known vegetables in this category are tomatoes and red peppers.

• Other vegetables are essentially white, at least under the skin. These include cauliflower, summer squash, potatoes, and radishes, many of which are good sources of vitamin C.

The Food Guide Pyramid recommends three to five daily servings of vegetables. One serving is one-half cup of any raw vegetable, except for lettuce and sprouts, which require one cup per serving. Because heating reduces water content, cooked vegetables require less space than uncooked vegetables and serving sizes may be smaller. Likewise, vegetable juices are more concentrated and require only one-half cup per serving.

Table 10.1

Sample Exchange Units Equivalent to One Serving

One grain serving

Cereals
1/4 c nugget cereals (Grape Nuts)
1/3 c concentrated bran cereals
1/2 c cooked hot cereal (oatmeal or Cream of Wheat)
3/4 c flaked cereals
1 1/2 c puffed cereals

Grains
1/4 c wheat germ
1/3 c brown or white rice
1/2 c pasta, macaroni, or noodles
1/2 c hominy, barley, or grits

Breads
1/2 bagel or English muffin
1 slice bread
1 piece pita bread
1 tortilla

Snacks
3/4 oz pretzels
3/4 oz rice cakes
4 crackers (1 oz)
3 c air-popped popcorn

One fruit serving

2 T raisins
3 dates
3 prunes
1/2 c grapes
3/4 c berries
1 apple
1 banana
1 peach
1 pear
3 apricots
1/2 grapefruit

3/4 c pineapple
2 kiwi
1/2 pomegranate
1/4 cantaloupe
1/4 papaya
1/4 melon
1/2 mango
5 kumquats
1 c honeydew
1 1/4 c strawberries
1 1/4 c watermelon

One dairy serving

1 oz low-fat cheese
1/4 c low-fat or nonfat cottage cheese
1/4 c part-skim ricotta cheese
1/4 c parmesan cheese

1/2 c evaporated skim milk
1 c nonfat or 1% milk
1 c low-fat or nonfat yogurt
1 c low-fat buttermilk

One meat serving

3 oz fish
3 oz poultry
3 oz meat (beef, poultry, lamb, etc.)
1 egg or 2 egg whites

1 T peanut butter
1/4 c cooked dry beans
1/4 c tuna
1/4 c tofu

One fat serving

1 t butter
1 T diet margarine
1 t mayonnaise
1 T diet mayonnaise
1 t oil
1 T salad dressing

2 T diet salad dressing
1 T cream cheese
2 T light cream cheese
2 T sour cream
4 T light sour cream
2 T coffee creamer (liquid)

It is a good idea to eat some vegetables raw and to steam or microwave vegetables for nutrient retention. Also, fresh and frozen vegetables have more nutritional value and are lower in sodium than canned vegetables.

Fruit

Fruits are also relatively low in calories, with just as much variety and nutritional value as vegetables. Essentially all fruit choices are high in carbohydrates and vitamins, and many provide excellent sources of fiber.

• Citrus fruits, such as oranges, grapefruit, and lemons, are loaded with vitamin C.

• Like orange-colored vegetables, orange fruits—including cantaloupe, apricots, and papaya—are rich in vitamin A and beta-carotene.

• Green fruits, such as honeydew melon and kiwi, and red fruits, such as strawberries and cherries, are also high in vitamin C.

• Yellow fruits—including peaches, mangos, and pineapples—are usually good sources of vitamin C.

• Fruits that are white, at least on the inside—including apples, pears, and bananas—are high in potassium.

• Dried fruit is particularly nutrient dense, and the natural sweetness makes it a healthy substitute for high-fat snacks such as candy bars. Raisins, dates, figs, and prunes are all superb energy sources, and prunes are the single best source of dietary fiber.

The Food Guide Pyramid recommends two to four servings of fruit every day. Table 10.1 presents sample exchange quantities for a variety of fruits. You will notice that one serving varies considerably depending upon the type of fruit eaten. For example, it takes one quarter of a melon or one-half of a grapefruit to equal three dates or two tablespoons of raisins. The difference is water content. Fresh fruit contains lots of water, whereas dried fruit is essentially a high-density carbohydrate. For people who prefer their fruit in liquid form, one-half cup of fruit juice equals one serving, but has less fiber than whole fruit.

Milk Products

The Food Guide Pyramid recommends two to three daily servings of low-fat dairy products, including milk, yogurt, and cheese. These foods are excellent sources of protein and calcium. Because whole milk products are high in fat, clients should be selective at the dairy counter. For example, skim milk, one-percent milk, low-fat yogurt, and nonfat cottage cheese offer heart-healthy alternatives to higher-fat dairy selections.

Refer to table 10.1 for exchange units equivalent to one dairy serving. Notice that one-quarter cup of low-fat cheese has similar nutritional value to one cup of one-percent milk. Although there are many sources of dietary protein, seniors may have difficulty obtaining sufficient calcium unless they regularly consume milk products. If clients have problems digesting milk (lactose intolerance), they should be sure to eat other foods that are high in calcium such as tofu, leafy greens, beans, broccoli, and sesame seeds.

Meats

This category includes meat, poultry, fish, eggs, nuts, and dry beans. All are good sources of protein, although some also contain significant amounts of fat. Table 10.2 presents sample foods in the meat category according to their fat content. Note that how meat is prepared has a lot to do with how much fat it provides. This nutritional aspect will be presented in more detail in the food preparation section.

While there are differences in fat content, protein exchange units are quite consistent among the foods in the meat category. As you can see from table 10.1, three ounces of meat, poultry, and fish (about the size of a deck of cards) have equal exchange value, as do one-quarter cup of dry beans and one-quarter cup of tuna. Encourage your clients to consume two to three servings, for a total of six to nine ounces, from the meat group on a daily basis.

Fats

The smallest section of the Food Guide Pyramid is the fat group, which should be consumed sparingly. Although all fats contain over nine calories per gram, some fats are more desirable than others from a health perspective. For example, consuming saturated fats (such as those found in mayonnaise, butter,

Table 10.2

Meat Group Foods Categorized by Fat Content

Low fat	Medium fat	High fat
All fish	Chicken with skin	Beef ribs
Egg whites	Turkey with skin	Pork ribs
Chicken without skin	Roast beef	Corned beef
Turkey without skin	Roast pork	Sausage
Venison	Roast lamb	Lunch meat
Rabbit	Veal cutlet	Ground pork
Top round	Ground beef	Hot dogs
Eye of round	Steaks	Fried chicken
Sirloin tenderloin	Canned salmon	Fried fish
Flank steak	Oil-packed tuna	Nuts
Veal	Whole eggs	Peanuts
Dry beans	Pork chops	Peanut butter

and sour cream) presents a higher risk for developing heart disease than polyunsaturated fats (such as those found in margarine and corn oil): There is evidence that monounsaturated fats (such as those in olive oil and canola oil) are even more desirable than polyunsaturated with respect to coronary health. See table 10.1 to determine serving equivalents for foods in the fat group.

As you are undoubtedly aware, fat consumption has become a major issue in mainstream America, with various authorities recommending different amounts of dietary fat intake. Whereas Dr. Dean Ornish (1993) advises that the heart patient eat only 10% of daily calories from fat, the American Heart Association and the American Dietetic Association allow up to 30% fat calories in the daily diet. According to the American Council on Exercise's *Personal Trainer Manual* (1996), most athletic individuals should consume between 20 to 30% of their calories from fat. We agree with this recommendation, but prefer diets closer to 20% fat calories.

> *An excellent diet plan for senior strength trainers is Dr. James Rippe's* Exercise Exchange Program *(Simon and Schuster Publishers), which provides about 23% fat, 23% protein, and 54% carbohydrate calories on a daily basis.*

Water: The Most Important Nutrient

Water is not included in the Food Guide Pyramid because it contains no calories and is not technically a food. Yet it is by far the most important human nutrient. The human body is mostly water (muscles are 80% water) and can survive only a few days without adequate hydration.

The standard recommendation is to consume eight 8-ounce glasses of water daily; people who exercise need considerably more. Unfortunately, the natural thirst mechanism declines with age, so have your clients monitor their water consumption to make sure they are well hydrated, drinking 10 to 12 glasses of water on exercise days.

Because coffee, tea, diet drinks, and alcoholic beverages act as diuretics (which have a dehydrating effect), your clients should not count these in their daily water supply; but they may substitute beverages such as seltzer and fruit juices for water. Apple juice is an excellent source of potassium, and orange juice is high in vitamin C. Cranberry juice is close to orange juice in vitamin C content and may help prevent bladder infections. Carrot juice is high in vitamin A, vitamin C, potassium, and fiber.

Three Steps to Better Nutrition

An eating program that provides all of the essential nutrients but limits fat consumption requires careful food selection, substitution, and preparation. The following suggestions should be useful to clients who want to implement more healthful eating habits.

Food Selection

If your clients follow the Food Guide Pyramid recommendations, emphasizing grains, vegetables, and fruit, along with moderate amounts of milk and meat products, their diets generally will be high in nutrition and low in fat. They should, however, be very selective in the fat category. Because saturated fats such as those found in butter, cream, egg yolks, palm oil, and coconut oil raise blood cholesterol levels, your clients should consume these food items sparingly. Instead, have them select monounsaturated fats (such as olive, canola, and peanut oils) or polyunsaturated fats (such as safflower, sunflower, and corn oils). While both mono- and polyunsaturated oils tend to lower blood cholesterol levels, monounsaturated oils may be preferred for reducing the risk of heart disease.

The following foods, as well as those shown in figure 10.2, contain less saturated fat than other choices in their category, and are preferred selections: fish; poultry without skin; low-fat milk, yogurt, and cottage cheese; olive, peanut, sunflower, safflower, corn, and canola oils.

> *Your clients should generally avoid prepared foods that contain saturated fats, such as palm and coconut oils, as well as hydrogenated products. These types of fats appear to be most detrimental in raising cholesterol levels, thereby increasing the risk of cardiovascular disease. The container label will indicate if a food is high in saturated fat or has been hydrogenated.*

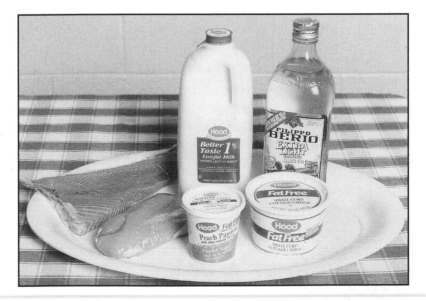

Figure 10.2 It is best to use low-fat fats and to substitute monounsaturated oils when possible.

Food Substitution

Most people have favorite foods they don't want to give up in spite of the fat content. The good news is that simple substitutions can reduce fat content without detracting from taste. For example, using evaporated skim milk in place of cream cuts fat and cholesterol content by more than 65%; and using plain non-fat yogurt or non-fat sour cream in place of sour cream on baked potatoes reduces cholesterol content by 90%—and supplies the body with twice as much beneficial calcium.

Other useful substitutes are two egg whites in place of a whole egg, herbs rather than table salt, low-fat frozen yogurt instead of ice cream, cocoa powder in place of chocolate squares in baked goods, and lemon juice or vinegar instead of high-fat salad dressings.

For clients with a sweet tooth, suggest dried fruit (raisins, dates, figs, prunes, dried apricots) in place of candy, cookies, and fat-rich baked goods. People who prefer crunchy snacks like potato chips may appreciate lower fat alternatives such as pretzels, baked chips, or carrot sticks.

Food Preparation

How food is prepared may increase or decrease the fat content. Frying can double and triple the calories in some foods. Using nonfat vegetable spray or a nonstick skillet can eliminate the fats and oils typically used for frying. It is also better to cook vegetables separate from meat, so they won't absorb fats from the meat. Suggest baked or broiled meats and steamed or microwaved vegetables for greatest retention of nutrients. Discourage seniors from adding butter and salt to vegetables during cooking—it takes less salt and fat to make food taste good after cooking than during cooking.

Energy for Exercise and Protein for Muscle Building

Your clients may be concerned about obtaining enough energy for their workouts and sufficient nutrients for building muscle. Although those who follow the Food Guide Pyramid recommendations should be well served in both areas, this section presents more specific information about the calorie and protein needs of senior strength trainers.

Strength training generally requires about 8 to 10 calories per minute during exercise performance (Wilmore et al. 1978). A client who completes a 25-minute circuit of resistance machines with little rest between successive exercises would therefore burn approximately 200 to 250 additional calories (Paffenbarger and Olsen 1996).

Because of its vigorous nature and anaerobic energy requirements, strength training leads to considerable postexercise calorie utilization. Resting metabolic rate may remain about 7% higher than normal for half a day after a demanding strength workout (Melby et al. 1993), burning an extra 50 to 75 calories.

In addition to these direct energy requirements, strength training produces more muscle and more active muscle—which consumes calories *all day long*. A pound of new muscle at rest apparently uses between 35 to 50 calories every 24 hours just for tissue maintenance (Campbell et al. 1994; Paffenbarger and Olsen 1996; Pratley et al. 1994). Since seniors typically add two to three pounds of lean (muscle) weight after two to three months of strength training (Campbell et al. 1994; Westcott and Guy 1996), the increase in resting metabolism due solely to more muscle may require an additional 75 to 100 calories per day, every day of the week.

Strength training may be responsible for a total of about 325 to 425 additional calories used on exercise days. This is consistent with the 15% increase in daily energy utilization experienced by the senior strength trainers in the landmark study at Tufts University (Campbell et al. 1994).

Based on these numbers, older adults who do strength training may eventually need to eat about 325 to 425 additional calories on exercise days and about 75 to 100 extra calories on nonexercise days to maintain their bodyweight. Although they can accomplish this by consuming high-energy drinks, sports bars, or other food supplements, they will do best to have additional servings from the Food Guide Pyramid. An extra serving each from the grains, fruits, vegetables, and milk groups should total about 325 to 425 calories and provide a variety of important nutrients. Of course, clients who want to lose bodyweight may maintain their usual food intake or even reduce their calories slightly.

Another concern among many strength training enthusiasts is obtaining sufficient protein to build more muscle tissue. Because muscle is 80% water, the more important factor is to maintain a high level of hydration, drinking at least eight glasses of water every day. Physically active individuals should drink two to four additional glasses of water on days when they exercise. Although it is also necessary to eat enough protein to facilitate muscle-building processes, the general protein recommendation of one gram per kilogram bodyweight appears to be optimal for senior strength trainers. Campbell et al. (1994) found no additional muscle-building benefit associated with extra protein in their senior strength training subjects, and an extensive research review by Williams (1993) did not reveal scientific evidence supporting protein supplementation.

Using the guideline of one gram of protein per kilogram of bodyweight, a senior female who weighs 130 pounds (about 60 kilograms) should consume approximately 60 grams of protein daily. A 180-pound (about 80 kilograms) senior male should eat approximately 80 grams of protein each day. For those who desire an extra margin of protein just to be sure, an additional serving of low-fat dairy products or lean meats should be more than adequate. Commercial protein supplements are generally unnecessary, but may be taken with a physician's or dietician's approval. Just be sure that extra protein is accompanied by extra water to facilitate kidney function. Discourage your clients from consuming excessive protein—too much protein can reduce body/bone calcium content and overstress the kidneys as they attempt to excrete the nitrogen waste products associated with protein metabolism.

Eating, Exercise, and Encouragement

Healthy eating is not the same as dieting. Dieting implies a significant reduction in calories for the purpose of losing weight, usually in a short period of time. Most weight-loss diets involve unnatural eating patterns and too few nutrients for optimum physical function. Because they are consuming reduced levels of important nutrients, most people cannot maintain these eating plans very long; and they typically regain the weight they have lost soon after they discontinue the diet.

Perhaps the most important thing you can do for overweight older clients is to provide sincere encouragement for desirable exercise and eating behavior. Help your clients set realistic short-term exercise and nutrition goals, and give plenty of positive reinforcement as they make progress in achieving them. An excellent resource in this area is Dr. Daniel Kosich's book Get Real: A Personal Guide to Real-Life Weight Management *(IDEA).*

Emphasize changes in body composition measurements rather than bodyweight, as strength trainers normally lose fat and add muscle at the same time. For example, a male client may add 4 pounds of lean weight and lose 8 pounds of fat weight during a 10-week training period. Although the bathroom scale shows only a 4-pound weight loss, the client has actually made a 12-pound change in body composition, which should be quite obvious in the way he looks and fits into his clothes.

Summary

Nutrition for senior strength trainers is basically the same as nutrition for all older adults who desire good health and body composition. Clients should find that a sound eating program provides plenty of energy for their strength training workouts, as well as sufficient protein and essential nutrients to enhance their muscle development. We recommend the food categories and portions presented in the United States Department of Agriculture Food Guide Pyramid: 6 to 11 daily servings of grains, 3 to 5 daily servings of vegetables, 2 to 4 daily servings of fruit, 2 to 3 daily servings of milk products, 2 to 3 daily servings of meats, and small quantities of fats such as nuts and monounsaturated oils.

Seniors who undertake strength training should drink about 10 to 12 glasses of water on their training days, and at least 8 glasses on nontraining days. Energy requirements for 25 minutes of circuit strength training may be 200 to 250 calories. The muscle-building effects of regular strength training may require an additional 325 to 425 calories on exercise days and 75 to 100 calories on nonexercise days. Although extra calories may be necessary for senior strength trainers to maintain their bodyweight, research does not reveal a need for extra protein (more than one gram of protein for each kilogram of bodyweight).

Senior exercise clients who want to lose body fat should find motivation in setting short-term goals and receiving positive reinforcement as they progress toward attainment of their goals.

Training Logs

Copy the following training logs for use with your clients. Copy at 145% to get 8.5" × 11" forms. Use Training Log 1 for 3-day-per-week workout programs and Training Log 2 for 4-day-per-week workout programs.

Training Log 1

Name _____

Order	Exercise	Reps / Sets	Set	Week # ___ Day 1			Day 2			Day 3			Week # ___ Day 1			Day 2			Day 3		
				1	2	3	1	2	3	1	2	3	1	2	3	1	2	3	1	2	3
1			Wt.																		
			Reps																		
2			Wt.																		
			Reps																		
3			Wt.																		
			Reps																		
4			Wt.																		
			Reps																		
5			Wt.																		
			Reps																		
6			Wt.																		
			Reps																		
7			Wt.																		
			Reps																		
8			Wt.																		
			Reps																		
9			Wt.																		
			Reps																		
10			Wt.																		
			Reps																		
11			Wt.																		
			Reps																		
Bodyweight																					
Date																					
Comments																					

Training Log 2

Name _____   Week # _____

Order	Upper body exercises	Reps		Day 1				Day 3			
		Sets	Set	1	2	3	4	1	2	3	4
1			Wt.								
			Reps								
2			Wt.								
			Reps								
3			Wt.								
			Reps								
4			Wt.								
			Reps								
5			Wt.								
			Reps								
6			Wt.								
			Reps								
7			Wt.								
			Reps								
	Bodyweight										
	Date										
	Comments										

Order	Lower body exercises	Reps		Day 2				Day 4			
		Sets	Set	1	2	3	4	1	2	3	4
1			Wt.								
			Reps								
2			Wt.								
			Reps								
3			Wt.								
			Reps								
4			Wt.								
			Reps								
5			Wt.								
			Reps								
6			Wt.								
			Reps								
	Bodyweight										
	Date										
	Comments										

References

Introduction

Campbell, W., Crim, M., Young, V., and W. Evans (1994). Increased energy requirements and changes in body composition with resistance training in older adults. *American Journal of Clinical Nutrition* 60:167-175.

Evans, W., and I. Rosenberg (1992). *Biomarkers*. New York: Simon and Schuster.

Fiatarone, M., Marks, E., Ryan, N., Meredith, C., Lipsitz, L., and W. Evans (1990). High-intensity strength training in nonagenarians. *Journal of the American Medical Association* 263(22):3029-3034.

Frontera, W., Meredith, C., O'Reilly, K., Knuttgen, H., and W. Evans (1988). Strength conditioning in older men: Skeletal muscle hypertrophy and improved function. *Journal of Applied Physiology* 64(3):1038-1044.

Hurley, B. (1994). Does strength training improve health status? *Strength and Conditioning Journal* 16:7-13.

Koffler, K., Menkes, A., Redmond, A., Whitehead, W., Pratley, R., and B. Hurley (1992). Strength training accelerates gastrointestinal transit in middle-aged and older men. *Medicine and Science in Sports and Exercise*: 24:415-419.

Menkes, A., Mazel, S., Redmond, R., Koffler, K., Libanati, C., Gunberg, C., Zizic, T. Hagberg, J., Pratley, R., and B. Hurley (1993). Strength training increases regional bone mineral density and bone remodeling in middle-aged and older men. *Journal of Applied Physiology* 74:2478-2484.

Nelson, M., Fiatarone, M., Morganti, C., Trice, I. Greenberg, R., and W. Evans (1994). Effects of high-intensity strength training on multiple risk factors for osteoporotic fractures. *Journal of the American Medical Association* 272(24):1909-1914.

Risch, S., Norvell, N., Pollock, M., Risch, E., Langer, H., Fulton, M., Graves, J., and S. Leggett (1993). Lumbar strengthening in chronic low back pain patients. *Spine* 18:232-238.

Tufts (1994). Never too late to build up your muscle. *Tufts University Diet and Nutrition Letter* 12:6-7.

Westcott, W. (1995). Keeping fit. *Nautilus* 4:2,4-5.

Westcott, W., and J. Guy (1996). A physical evolution: Sedentary adults see marked improvements in as little as two days a week. *IDEA Today* 14(9):58-65.

Chapter 1

American Association of Cardiovascular and Pulmonary Rehabilitation (1995). *Guidelines for Cardiac Rehabilitation Programs*. 2d ed. Champaign, IL: Human Kinetics.

American College of Sports Medicine (1991). *Guidelines for Exercise Testing and Prescription* (4th Edition). Philadelphia: Lea & Febiger.

Ballor, D., Katch, V., Becque, M., and C. Marks (1988). Resistance weight training during caloric restriction enhances lean body weight maintenance. *American Journal of Clinical Nutrition* 47:19-25.

Bell, N., Godsen, R., and D. Henry (1988). The effects of muscle-building exercise on vitamin D and mineral metabolism. *Journal of Bone Mineral Research* 3:369-373.

Blessing, D., Stone, M., and R. Byrd (1987). Blood lipid and hormonal changes from jogging and weight training of middle-aged men. *Journal of Applied Sports Science Research* 1:25-29.

Blumenthal, J., Siegel, W., and M. Appelbaum (1991). Failure of exercise to reduce blood pressure in patients with mild hypertension. *Journal of the American Medical Association* 266:2098-2101.

Boyden, T., Pamenter, R., Going, S., Lohman, T., Hall, M., Houtkooper, L., Bunt, J., Ritenbaugh, C., and M. Aickin (1993). Resistance exercise training is associated with decreases in serum low-density lipoprotein cholesterol levels in premenopausal women. *Archives of Internal Medicine* 153:97-100.

Brehm, B., and B. Keller (1990). Diet and exercise factors that influence weight and fat loss. *IDEA Today* 8:33-46.

Butler, R., Beierwaltes, W., and F. Rogers (1987). The cardiovascular response to circuit weight training in patients with cardiac disease. *Journal of Cardiopulmonary Rehabilitation* 7:402-409.

Butts, N., and S. Price (1994). Effects of a 12-week weight training program on the body composition of women over 30 years of age. *Journal of Strength and Conditioning Research* 8(4):265-269.

Campbell, W., Crim, M., Young, V., and W. Evans (1994). Increased energy requirements and changes in body composition with resistance training in older adults. *American Journal of Clinical Nutrition* 60:167-175.

Colletti, L., Edwards, J., Gordon, L., Shary, J., and N. Bell (1989). The effects of muscle-building exercise on bone mineral density of the radius, spine and hip in young men. *Calcified Tissue International.* 45:12-14.

Cordain, L., Latin, R., and J. Behnke (1986). The effects of an aerobic running program on bowel transit time. *Journal of Sports Medicine* 26:101-104.

Council On Exercise Of The American Diabetes Association (1990). Technical review: Exercise and NIDDM. *Diabetes Care* 13:785-789.

Craig, B., Everhart, J., and R. Brown (1989). The influence of high-resistance training on glucose tolerance in young and elderly subjects. *Mechanisms of Ageing and Development* 49:147-157.

Durak, E. (1989). Exercise for specific populations: Diabetes mellitus. *Sports Training, Medicine and Rehabilitation* 1:175-180.

Durak, E., Jovanovis-Peterson, L., and C. Peterson (1990). Randomized crossover study of effect of resistance training on glycemic control, muscular strength, and cholesterol in type I diabetic men. *Diabetes Care* 13:1039-1042.

Eriksson, J., Taimela, S., Eriksson, K., Parviainen, S., Peltonen, J., and U. Kujala (1997). Resistance training in the treatment of non-insulin dependent diabetes mellitus. *International Journal of Sports Medicine* 18(4):242-246.

Evans, W., and I. Rosenberg (1992). *Biomarkers.* New York: Simon and Schuster.

Faigenbaum, A., Skrinar, W., Cesare, W., Kraemer, W., and H. Thomas (1990). Physiologic and symptomatic responses of cardiac patients to resistance exercise. *Archives of Physical Medicine and Rehabilitation* 70:395-398.

Fiatarone, M., Marks, E., Ryan, N., Meredith, C. Lipsitz, L., and W. Evans (1990). High-intensity strength training in nonagenarians. *Journal of the American Medical Association* 263(22):3029-3034.

Frontera, W., Meredith, C., O'Reilly, K., Knuttgen, H., and W. Evans (1988). Strength conditioning in older men: Skeletal muscle hypertrophy and improved function. *Journal of Applied Physiology* 64(3):1038-1044.

Ghilarducci, L., Holly, R., and E. Amsterdam (1989). Effects of high resistance training in coronary heart disease. *American Journal of Cardiology* 64:866-870.

Gillette, C., Bullough, R., and C. Melby (1994). Postexercise energy expenditure in response to acute aerobic or resistive exercise. *International Journal of Sport Nutrition* 4:347-360.

Goldberg, L., Elliot, L., Schultz, R., and F. Kloste (1984). Changes in lipid and lipoprotein levels after weight training. *Journal of the American Medical Association* 252:504-506.

Grimby, G., Aniansson, A., Hedberg, M., Henning, G., Granguard, U., and H. Kvist (1992). Training can improve muscle strength and endurance in 78 to 84 year old men. *Journal of Applied Physiology* 73:2517-2523.

Haennel, R., Quinney, H., and C. Kappagoda (1991). Effects of hydraulic circuit training following coronary artery bypass surgery. *Medicine and Science in Sports and Exercise* 23:158-165.

Harris, K., and R. Holly (1987). Physiological response to circuit weight training in borderline hypertensive subjects. *Medicine and Science in Sports and Exercise* 10:246-252.

Hurley, B. (1994). Does strength training improve health status? *Strength and Conditioning Journal* 16:7-13.

Hurley, B., Hagberg, J., Goldberg, A., Seals, D., Ehsani, A., Brennan, R., and J. Holloszy (1988). Resistive training can reduce coronary risk factors without altering VO$_2$ max or percent body fat. *Medicine and Science in Sports and Exercise* 20:150-154.

Johnson, C., Stone, M., Lopez, S., Hebert, J., Kilgoe, L., and R. Byrd (1982). Diet and exercise in middle-aged men. *Journal of the Dietetic Association* 81:695-701.

Jones, A., Pollock, M., Graves, J., Fulton, M., Jones, W., MacMillan, M., Baldwin, D., and J. Cirulli (1988). *Safe, specific testing and rehabilitative exercise for muscles of the lumbar spine.* Santa Barbara, California: Sequoia Communications.

Katz, J., and B. Wilson (1992). The effects of a six-week, low-intensity Nautilus circuit training program on resting blood pressure in females. *The Journal of Sports Medicine and Physical Fitness* 32:299-302.

Kelemen, M., Stewart, K., Gillilan, R., Ewart, C., Valenti, S., Manley, J., and M. Kelemen (1986). Circuit weight training in cardiac patients. *Journal of the American College of Cardiology* 7:38-42.

Kelly, G. (1997). Dynamic resistance exercise and resting blood pressure in healthy adults: a meta-analysis. *Journal of Applied Physiology* 82:1559-1565.

Koffler, K., Menkes, A., Redmond, A., Whitehead, W., Pratley, R., and B. Hurley (1992). Strength training accelerates gastrointestinal transit in middle-aged and older men. *Medicine and Science in Sports and Exercise* 24:415-419.

Kokkinos, P., Hurley, B., Vaccaro, P., Patterson, J., Gardner, L., Ostrove, S., and A. Goldberg (1988). Effects of low- and high-repetition resistive training on lipoprotein-lipid profiles. *Medicine and Science in Sports and Exercise* 20:50-54.

Kokkinos, P., Hurley, B., Smutok, M., Farmer, C., Reece, C., Shulman, R., Charabogos, C., Patterson, J., Will, S., DeVane-Bell, J., and A. Goldberg (1991). Strength training does not improve lipoprotein lipid profiles in men at risk for CHD. *Medicine and Science in Sports and Exercise* 23:1134-1139.

Kraemer, W. and S. Fleck (1997). Strength training for seniors. *Strength and Health Report* 1 (15):1-2.

Lohmann, D. and F. Liebold (1978). Diminished insulin responses in highly trained athletes. *Metabolism* 27 (5):521-523.

Marks, R. (1993). The effect of isometric quadriceps strength training in mid-range for osteoarthritis of the knee. *Arthritis Care Research* 6:52-56.

McCartney, N., Hicks, A., Martin, J., and C. Webber (1996). A longitudinal trial of weight training in the elderly—continued improvements in year two. *Journals of Gerontology Series A—Biological Sciences and Medical Sciences* 51(6):B425-B433.

Melby, C., Scholl, C., Edwards, G., and R. Bullough (1993). Effect of acute resistance exercise on postexercise energy expenditure and resting metabolic rate. *Journal of Applied Physiology* 75(4):1847-1853.

Menkes, A., Mazel, S., Redmond, R., Koffler, K., Libanati, C., Gundberg, C., Zizic, T., Hagberg, J., Pratley, R., and B. Hurley (1993). Strength training increases regional bone mineral density and bone remodeling in middle-aged and older men. *Journal of Applied Physiology* 74:2478-2484.

Miller, W., Sherman, W., and J. Ivy (1984). Effect of strength training on glucose tolerance and post glucose insulin response. *Medicine and Science in Sports and Exercise* 16(6):539-543.

Morrow, J. (1997). Relationship of low back pain to exercise habits. Paper presented at American College of Sports Medicine Conference, Denver, Colorado, May 31.

Nelson, M., Fiatarone, M., Morganti, C., Trice, I., Greenberg, R., and W. Evans (1994). Effects of high-intensity strength training on multiple risk factors for osteoporotic fractures. *Journal of the American Medical Association* 272(24):1909-1914.

Notelovitz, M., Martin, D., Tesar, R., Khan, F., Probart, C., Fields, C., and L. McKenzie (1991). Estrogen therapy and variable resistance weight training increase bone mineral in surgically menopausal women. *Journal of Bone Mineral Research* 6:583-590.

Paffenbarger, R., and E. Olsen (1996). *Life fit: An effective exercise program for optimal health and a longer life.* Champaign, IL: Human Kinetics.

Pratley, R., Nicklas, B., Rubin, M., Miller, J., Smith, A., Smith, M., Hurley, B., and A. Goldberg. (1994). Strength training increases resting metabolic rate and norepinephrine levels in healthy 50 to 65 year-old men. *Journal of Applied Physiology* 76:133-137.

Quirk, A., Newman, R., and K. Newman (1985). An evaluation of interferential therapy, shortwave diathermy and exercise in the treatment of osteo-arthritis of the knee. *Physiotherapy* 71:55-57.

Risch, S., Nowell, N., Pollock, M., Risch, E., Langer, H., Fulton, M., Graves, J., and S. Leggett (1993). Lumbar strengthening in chronic low back pain patients. *Spine* 18:232-238.

Ryan, A., Treuth, M., Rubin, M., Miller, J., Nicklas, B., Landis, D., Pratley, R., Libanati, C., Grundberg, C., and B. Hurley (1994). Effects of strength training on bone mineral density: hormonal and bone turnover relationships. *Journal of Applied Physiology* 77:1678-1684.

Singh, N., Clements, K., and M. Fiatarone (1997). A randomized controlled trial of progressive resistance training in depressed elders. *Journal of Gerontology* 52A(1):M27-M35.

Smutok, M., Reece, C., Kokkinos, P., Farmer, C., Dawson, P., Shulman, R., DeVane-Bell, J., Patterson, J., Charabogos, C., Goldley, A., and B. Hurley (1993). Aerobic vs. strength training for risk factor intervention in middle-aged men at high risk for coronary heart disease. *Metabolism* 42:177-184.

Snow-Harter, C., Bouxsein, M., Lewis, B., Carter, D., and R. Marcus (1992). Effects of resistance and endurance exercise on bone mineral status of young women: A randomized exercise intervention trial. *Journal of Bone Mineral Research* 7:761-769.

Stewart, K., Mason, M., and M. Kelemen (1988). Three-year participation in circuit weight training improves muscular strength and self-efficacy in cardiac patients. *Journal of Cardiopulmonary Rehabilitation* 8:292-296.

Stone, M., Blessing, D., Byrd, R., Tew, J., and D. Boatwright (1982). Physiological effects of a short term resistive training program on middle-aged untrained men. *National Strength and Conditioning Association Journal* 4:16-20.

Taunton, J., Martin, A., Rhodes, E., Wolski, L., Donnelly, M., and J. Elliot (1997). Exercise for older women: Choosing the right prescription. *British Journal of Sports Medicine* 31:5-10.

Tufts University Diet and Nutrition Letter (1992). An IQ test for losers. 10(March):6-7.

Tufts University Diet and Nutrition Letter. (1994) Never too late to build up your muscle. 12(September):6-7.

Ulrich, I., Reid, C., and R. Yeater (1987). Increased HDL-cholesterol levels with a weight training program. *Southern Medical Journal* 80:328-331.

Vander, L., Franklin, B., Wrisley, D., and M. Rubenfire (1986). Acute cardiovascular responses to Nautilus exercise in cardiac patients: Implications for exercise training. *Annals of Sports Medicine* 2:165-169.

Westcott, W. (1986). Strength training and blood pressure. *American Fitness Quarterly* 5: 38-39.

Westcott, W. (1995). Keeping fit. *Nautilus* 4(2):5-7.

Westcott, W. (1997). Golf and strength training are compatible activities. Paper presented at IDEA World Research Forum, Anaheim, California, July 23.

Westcott, W., and B. Howes (1983). Blood pressure response during weight training exercise. *National Strength and Conditioning Association Journal* 5:67-71.

Westcott, W., and J. Guy (1996). A physical evolution: Sedentary adults see marked improvements in as little as two days a week. *IDEA Today* 14(9):58-65.

Westcott, W., Dolan, F., and T. Cavicchi (1996). Golf and strength training are compatible activities. *Journal of Strength and Conditioning* 18(4):54-56.

Wilmore, J., Parr, R., Vodak, P., and T. Barstow (1976). Strength, endurance, BMR, and body composition changes with circuit weight training. *Medicine and Science in Sports and Exercise* 8:59-60.

Chapter 2

American College of Sports Medicine (1990). The recommended quantity and quality of exercise for developing and maintaining cardiorespiratory and muscular fitness in healthy adults. *Medicine and Science in Sports and Exercise* 22:265-274.

Baechle, T., and B. Groves (1998). *Weight training: Steps to success.* Champaign, IL: Human Kinetics.

Baechle, T., and R. Earle (1995). *Fitness Weight Training.* Champaign, IL: Human Kinetics.

Braith, R., Graves, J., Pollock, M., Leggett, S., Carpenter, D., and A. Colvin (1989). Comparison of two versus three days per week of variable resistance training during 10 and 18 week programs. *International Journal of Sports Medicine* 10:450-454.

DeMichele, P., Pollock, M., Graves, J., Foster, D., Carpenter, D., Garzarella, L., Brechue, W., and M. Fulton. (1997). Isometric torso rotation strength: Effect of training frequency on its development. *Archives of Physical Medicine and Rehabilitation* 78:64-69.

Faigenbaum, A., Zaichkowsky, J., Westcott, W., Micheli, L., and A. Fehlandt (1993). The effects of a twice-a-week strength training program on children. *Pediatric Exercise Science* 5:339-346.

Faigenbaum, A., Westcott, W., Micheli, L., Outerbridge, A., Long, C., LaRosa-Loud, R., and L. Zaichkowsky (1996). The effects of strength training and detraining on children. *Journal of Strength and Conditioning Research* 10(2):109-114.

Fiatarone, M., Marks, E., Ryan, N., Meredith, C., Lipsitz, A., and W. Evans (1990). High-intensity strength training in nonagenarians. *Journal of the American Medical Association* 263(22):3029-3034.

Fleck, S., and W. Kraemer (1997). *Designing resistance training programs. 2nd Edition.* Champaign, IL: Human Kinetics.

Frontera, W., Meredith, C., O'Reilly, K., Knuttgen, H., and W. Evans (1988). Strength conditioning in older men: Skeletal muscle hypertrophy and improved function. *Journal of Applied Physiology* 64(3):1038-1044.

Kraemer, W., Purvis, T., and W. Westcott (1996). Everything you wanted to know about strength training. *IDEA Personal Trainer* 7(6):20-22.

Miles, M., Li, Y., Rinard, J., Clarkson, P., and J. Williamson (1997). Eccentric exercise augments the cardiovascular response to static exercise. *Medicine and Science in Sports and Exercise* 29:457-466.

Nelson, M., Fiatarone, M., Morganti, C., Trice, I., Greenberg, R., and W. Evans 1994. Effects of high-intensity strength training on multiple risk factors for osteoporotic fractures. *Journal of the American Medical Association* 272(24):1909-1914.

Stadler, L., Stubbs, N., and M. Vukovich (1997). A comparison of a 2-day and 3-day per week resistance training program on strength gains in older adults (abstract). *Medicine and Science in Sports and Exercise* 29:S254.

Starkey, D., Pollock, M., Ishida, Y., Welsch, M., Brechue, W., Graves, J., and M. Feigenbaum (1996). Effects of resistance training volume on strength and muscle thickness. *Medicine and Science in Sports and Exercise* 28(10):1311-1320.

Westcott, W. (1995). *Strength fitness: Physiological principles and training techniques.* 4th ed. Dubuque, Iowa: Brown and Benchmark.

Westcott, W., Greenberger, K., and D. Milius (1989). Strength training research: Sets and repetitions. *Scholastic Coach* 58:98-100.

Westcott, W., and J. Guy (1996). A physical evolution. *IDEA Today* 14(9):58-65.

Chapter 3

Graves, J., Pollock, M., Jones, A., Colvin, A., and S. Leggett (1989). Specificity of limited range of motion variable resistance training. *Medicine and Science in Sports and Exercise* 21(1):84-89.

Jones, A., Pollock, M., Graves, J., Fulton, M., Jones, W., MacMillan, M., Baldwin, D., and J. Cirulli (1988). *Safe, specific testing and rehabilitative exercise for the muscles of the lumbar spine.* Santa Barbara, California: Sequoia Communications.

Risch, S., Nowell, M., Pollock, M., Risch, E., Langer, H., Fulton, M., Graves, J., and S. Leggett (1993). Lumbar strengthening in chronic low back pain patients. *Spine* 18:232-238.

Westcott, W. (1995a). Transformation: How to take them from sedentary to active. *IDEA Today* 13:7,46-54.

Westcott, W. (1995b). Strength training for life: Keeping fit. *Nautilus* 4:2, 5-7.

Westcott, W., Dolan, F., and T. Cavicchi (1996). Golf and strength training are compatible activities. *Strength and Conditioning* 18(4):54-56.

Recommended Reading

Baechle, T., and R. Earle (1995). *Fitness Weight Training.* Champaign, IL: Human Kinetics.

Baechle, T., and B. Groves (1998). *Weight Training: Steps To Success.* Champaign, IL: Human Kinetics.

Dishman, R. (1988). *Exercise Adherence.* Champaign, IL. Human Kinetics.

Wilmore, J., and D. Costill (1994). *Physiology of Sport and Exercise.* Champaign, IL: Human Kinetics.

Chapter 4

Penn State Sports Medicine Newsletter (1997). Rating pain. 5(10):6.

Chapter 5

Westcott, W. (1995). Keeping fit. *Nautilus* 4:2,4-5.

Recommended Reading

Westcott, W. (1995a). *Strength fitness: Physiological principles and training.* 4th ed. Dubuque, Iowa: Brown and Benchmark.

Westcott, W. (1995b). Transformation: How to take them from sedentary to active. *IDEA Today* 13:7,46-54.

Chapter 6

Baechle, T., and R. Earle (1995). *Fitness Weight Training*. Champaign, IL: Human Kinetics.

Chapter 7

Recommended Reading

American Health (1994). A go-anywhere resistance-band workout. *American Health* 13:4,42.

Davis, J. (1997). Flexible fitness option: body-sculpting bands great for people on the go. *Chicago Sun-Times* (October 22).

Horn, D. (1996). Elastic bands can be an affordable way to strengthen muscles. *Houston Chronicle* (July 7).

McNaghten, M. (1993). A rubber band workout. *New Woman* 23:6,142.

Purvis, T. (1997). Totally tubular: The science behind elastic resistance. *Idea Today* 15:10,44-51.

SPRI Products (1990). *Rubber band advantage*. Wheeling, IL: SPRI Products. Video.

Wolfram, C. (1997). Dynaband dynamite for senior exercise. *New Orleans Times-Picayune* (Feb 2).

Zook, S. (1987). *The rubber band shape-up program*. Phoenix: ORTHO-SPORT Publi-cations.

Chapter 8

Dishman, R. (1988). *Exercise Adherence*. Champaign, IL: Human Kinetics.

Girouard, C., and B. Hurley (1995). Does strength training inhibit gains in range of motion from flexibility training in older adults? *Medicine and Science in Sports and Exercise* 27(10):1444-1449.

Golding, L., Myers, C., and W. Sinning (1989). *Y's Way To Physical Fitness*. Champaign, IL: Human Kinetics.

Westcott, W. (1987). *Building Strength at the YMCA*. Champaign, IL: Human Kinetics.

Westcott, W. (1994). Strength training for life: Weightloads: Go figure. *Nautilus Magazine* Fall 3(4):5-7.

Westcott, W. (1995). Strength training for life: Keeping fit. *Nautilus Magazine* Spring 4(2):5-7.

Westcott, W. (1996). *Building Strength and Stamina*. Champaign, IL: Human Kinetics.

Westcott, W., Dolan, F., and T. Cavicchi (1996). Golf and strength training are compatible activities. *Strength and Conditioning* 18(4):54-56.

Recommended Reading

National Institutes of Health Technology Assessment Conference Statement (1994). Bioelectri-cal impedance analysis in body composition measurement. (December 12-14). Washington, D.C.

Chapter 9

American Association of Cardiovascular and Pulmonary Rehabilitation (1995). *Guidelines for Cardiac Rehabilitation Programs*. 2d ed. Champaign, IL: Human Kinetics.

Arthritis Foundation (1997). Arthritis fact sheet. Atlanta.

Borg, G. (1998). *Borg's Perceived Exertion and Pain Scales*. Champaign, IL: Human Kinetics.

Campbell, W., Crim, M., Young, V., and W. Evans (1994). Increased energy requirements and changes in body composition with resistance training in older adults. *American Journal of Clinical Nutrition* 60:167-175.

Clark, J. (1997). Programming for adults with age-related health challenges. *American Council On Exercise Certified News* 3(5):4-6.

Drought, J. (1995). Resistance exercise in cardiac rehabilitation. *Strength and Conditioning* 17(2):56-64.

Eriksson, J., Taimela, S., Eriksson, K., Parviainen, S., Peltonen, J., and U. Kujala (1997). Resistance training in the treatment of non-insulin dependent diabetes mellitus. *International Journal of Sports Medicine* 18(4):242-246.

Evans, W., and I. Rosenberg (1992). *Biomarkers*. New York: Simon and Schuster.

Faigenbaum, A., Skrinar, G., Cesare, W., Kraemer, W., and H. Thomas (1990). Physiologic and symptomatic responses of cardiac patients to resistance exercise. *Archives of Physical Medicine and Rehabilitation* 70:395-398.

Faigenbaum, A., Zaichkowsky, L., Westcott, W., Lang, C., LaRosa-Loud, R., Micheli, L., and A. Outerbridge (1997). Psychological effects of strength training on children. *Journal of Sport Behavior* 20(2):164-175.

Fiatarone, M., Marks, E., Ryan, N., Meredith, C., Lipsitz, L., and W. Evans (1990). High-intensity strength training in nonagenarians. *Journal of the American Medical Association* 263(22):3029-3034.

Foltz-Gray, D. (1997). Bully the pain. *Arthritis Today* (July-August):18-25.

Foreman, J. (1997). A big, bad, ugly disease. *The Boston Globe* (August 4). Boston, Massachusetts.

Frontera, W., Meredith, C., O'Reilly, K., Knuttgen, H., and W. Evans (1988). Strength conditioning in older men: Skeletal muscle hypertrophy and improved function. *Journal of Applied Physiology* 64(3):1038-1044.

Ghilarducci, L., Holly, R., and E. Amsterdam (1989). Effects of high resistance training in coronary heart disease. *American Journal of Cardiology* 64:866-870.

Hargrove, T. (1996). Study: Nearly 75 percent in United States are overweight. *The Patriot Ledger* (November 26). Quincy, Massachusetts.

Hughes, V., Frontera, W., Dallal, G., Lutz, K., Fisher, E., and W. Evans (1995). Muscle strength and body composition: Associations with bone density in older subjects. *Medicine and Science In Sports and Exercise* 7(27):967-974.

Jones, A., Pollock, M., Graves, J., Fulton, M., Jones, W., MacMillan, M., Baldwin, D., and J. Cirulli (1988). *Safe, specific testing and rehabilitative exercise for muscles of the lumbar spine*. Santa Barbara, California: Sequoia Communications.

Kelemen, M., Stewart, K., Gillilan, R., Ewart, C., Valenti, S., Manley, J., and M. Keleman (1986). Circuit weight training in cardiac patients. *Journal of the American College of Cardiology* 7:38-42.

Menkes, A., Mazel, S., Redmond, R., Koffler, K., Libanati, C., Gunberg, C., Zizic, T., Hagberg, J., Pratley, R., and B. Hurley (1993). Strength training increases regional bone mineral density and bone remodeling in middle-aged and older men. *Journal of Applied Physiology* 74:2478-2484.

Nelson, M., Fiatarone, M., Morganti, C., Trice, I., Greenberg, R., and W. Evans (1994). Effects of high-intensity strength training on multiple risk factors for osteoporotic fractures. *Journal of the American Medical Association* 272(24):1909-1914.

President's Council on Physical Fitness and Sports Research Digest (1997). Physical activity and the prevention of Type II (non-insulin dependent) diabetes. 2(10):5.

Rimmer, J. (1997). Programming: Exercise guidelines for special medical populations. *IDEA Today* 15(5):26-34.

Risch, S., Norvell, N., Pollock, M., Risch, E., Langer, H., Fulton, M., Graves, J., and S. Leggett (1993). Lumbar strengthening in chronic low back pain patients. *Spine* 18:232-238.

Singh, N., Clements, K., and M. Fiatarone (1997). A randomized controlled trial of progressive resistance training in depressed elders. *Journal of Gerontology* 52A(1):M27-M35.

Tufts University Diet and Nutrition Letter (1994). Never too late to build up your muscle. 12(September):6-7

Vander, L., Franklin, B., Wrisley, D., and M. Rubenfire (1986). Acute cardiovascular response to circuit weight training in patients with cardiac disease. *Annals of Sports Medicine* 2:165-169.

Weil, R. (1993). Mall walking can provide exercise, companionship, first chance at sales. *Diabetes In The News* 12(1):58-59.

Westcott, W. (1995). Keeping fit. *Nautilus* 4(2):5-7.

Westcott, W., and J. Guy (1996). A physical evolution: Sedentary adults see marked improvements in as little as two days a week. *IDEA Today* 14(9):58-65.

Westcott, W., Dolan, F., and T. Cavicchi (1996). Golf and strength training are compatible activities. *Journal of Strength and Conditioning* 18(4):54-56.

Westcott, W., and S. O'Grady (1998). Strength training and cardiac postrehab. *IDEA Personal Trainer*, 9(2):41-6.

Chapter 10

American Council on Exercise (1996). *Personal Trainer Manual, Second Edition.* San Diego: American Council on Exercise.

Campbell, W., Crim, M., Young, V., and W. Evans (1994). Increased energy requirements and changes in body composition with resistance training in older adults. *American Journal of Clinical Nutrition* 60:167-175.

Hargrove, T. (1996). Study: Nearly 75 percent in United States are overweight. *The Patriot Ledger* (November 26). Quincy, Massachusetts.

Kosich, D. (1995). *Get Real: A Personal Guide To Real Life Weight Management.* San Diego: IDEA.

Melby, C., Scholl, C., Edwards, G., and R. Bullough (1993). Effect of acute resistance exercise on postexercise energy expenditure and resting metabolic rate. *Journal of Applied Physiology.* 75(4):1847-1853.

Ornish, D. (1993). *Eat more, weigh less: Dr. Dean Ornish's life choice program for losing weight safely while eating abundantly.* New York: Harper Collins.

Paffenbarger, R., and E. Olsen (1996). *Lifefit: An effective exercise program for optimal health and a longer life.* Champaign, IL: Human Kinetics.

Pratley, R., Nicklas, B., Rubin, M., Miller, J., Smith, A., Smith, M., Hurley, B., and A. Goldberg (1994). Strength training increases resting metabolic rate and norepinephrine levels in healthy 50- to 65-year-old men. *Journal of Applied Physiology.* 76:133-137.

Rippe, J. (1992). *The exercise exchange program.* New York: Simon and Schuster.

Westcott, W., and J. Guy (1996). A physical evolution: Sedentary adults see marked improvements in as little as two days a week. *IDEA Today* 14(9):58-65.

Williams, M. (1993). Nutritional supplements for strength trained athletes. *Sports Science Exchange* 6(6):1-4.

Wilmore, J., Parr, R., Ward, P., Vodak, P., Barstow, T., Pipes, T., Grimditch, G., and P. Leslie (1978). Energy cost of circuit weight training. *Medicine and Science in Sports.* 10:75-78.

Recommended Reading

American Heart Association (1989). *Low-fat, Low-cholesterol Cookbook.* New York: Random House.

Index

About the Authors

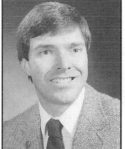

With more than 35 years in strength training as an athlete, coach, teacher, professor, researcher, writer, and speaker, **Wayne Westcott**, PhD, is recognized as a leading authority on fitness. He has served as a strength training consultant for numerous organizations and programs, including Nautilus, the President's Council on Physical Fitness and Sports, the National Sports Performance Association, the International Association of Fitness Professionals (IDEA), the American Council on Exercise, the YMCA of the USA, and the National Youth Sports Safety Foundation. He was awarded the IDEA Lifetime Achievement Award in 1993 and was honored with a Healthy American Fitness Leader Award in 1995.

Westcott is currently the fitness research director at the South Shore YMCA in Quincy, Massachusetts, where he has carefully studied the physiological responses of adults to various programs of strength exercise. In 1996 he conducted a landmark study of 1,132 subjects showing that men and women over age 50 build strength and develop muscle at the same rate as younger adults. Together with co-author Tom Baechle, he wrote *Strength Training Past 50*, which was ranked as one of the ten best health and fitness books of 1997.

Westcott has authored ten other books on strength training, including *Building Strength and Stamina* and *Strength Fitness: Physiological Principles and Training Techniques*. He has published over 300 articles in professional fitness journals and has written a weekly fitness column for one of Boston's largest newspapers since 1986. He has served on the editorial boards of *Prevention, Shape, Men's Health, Fitness, Club Industry, American Fitness Quarterly*, and *Nautilus*.

Westcott lives in Abington, Massachusetts, with his wife, Claudia. He enjoys strength training, running, cycling, and gardening.

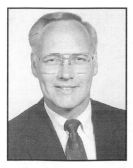

As an exercise leader for 16 years at the Creighton University Cardiac Rehabilitation program (one of the earliest to include a bona fide strength training component), **Thomas R. Baechle**, EdD, has a great deal of practical experience working with the over 50 population. He also has more than 20 years' experience teaching weight training and strength training for athletes at the college level. He currently serves as chair of the exercise science department at Creighton University, where his honors include an Excellence in Teaching Award.

Baechle is the executive director of the NSCA Certification Commission, the certifying body for the National Strength and Conditioning Association (NSCA), and is president of the National Organization for Competency Assurance, an international organization that sets quality standards for credentialing organizations. He has earned credentials from the NSCA's Certification Commission as a Certified Strength and Conditioning Specialist and Certified Personal Trainer; from the American College of Sports Medicine as a Test Technologist and Exercise Specialist; and from the United States Weightlifting Federation as a Level 1 Weightlifting Coach. He is cofounder, past president, and former director of education for NSCA, and in 1998 he received the organization's Lifetime Achievement Award.

Baechle has authored seven previous strength training texts, including the highly popular *Fitness Weight Training*. He also served as editor for NSCA's *Essentials of Strength Training and Conditioning*, a comprehensive text that has contributed to the growing number of university-level courses that prepare professionals for careers in strength and conditioning. Three of Baechle's texts have been translated into French or Japanese.

Baechle lives in Omaha, Nebraska, with his wife Susan and two sons, Todd and Clark. He enjoys strength training, woodworking, and making crafts.

More Resources from Westcott and Baechle

Essentials of Strength Training and Conditioning
National Strength and Conditioning Association
Thomas R. Baechle, EdD, CSCS, Editor
1994 • Hardcover • 560 pp • Item BNSC0694 • ISBN 0-87322-694-1 • $49.00 ($72.95 Canadian)

Weight Training
Steps to Success (Second Edition)
Thomas R. Baechle, EdD, CSCS, NSCA-CPT, and Barney R. Groves, PhD, CSCS
1998 • Paper • 192 pp • Item PBAE0718 • ISBN 0-88011-718-4 • $15.95 ($22.95 Canadian)

Weight Training Video
Steps to Success (57-minute videotape)
1993 • Item MBAE0243 • ISBN 0-87322-485-X • $29.95 ($44.95 Canadian)

Weight Training Instruction
Steps to Success
Thomas R. Baechle, EdD, CSCS, and Barney R. Groves, PhD, CSCS
1994 • Paper • 208 pp • Item PBAE0618 • ISBN 0-87322-618-6 • $19.95 ($29.95 Canadian)

Building Strength and Stamina
New Nautilus Training for Total Fitness
Wayne Westcott, PhD/Nautilus International
1996 • Paper • 248 pp • Item PWES0550 • ISBN 0-88011-550-5 • $16.95 ($24.95 Canadian)

Fitness Weight Training
Thomas R. Baechle, EdD, CSCS, and Roger Earle, MA, CSCS
1995 • Paper • 176 pp • Item PBAE0445 • ISBN 0-87322-445-0 • $15.95 ($21.95 Canadian)

Human Kinetics
The Information Leader in Physical Activity

1 2 4 0